52 SMALL CHANGES
FOR THE FAMILY

52
SMALL
CHANGES
for the
FAMILY

BRETT BLUMENTHAL
DANIELLE SHEA TAN

CHRONICLE BOOKS
SAN FRANCISCO

To my family—David, Alexander, Mom, Bill, Philip, and Leslie.
All of you are cherished and so greatly appreciated for all you do
to support me. I love you.

— B. B.

To my boys—Erol, Evren, and Aydin—you are my everything.
Your sacrifices to make this book happen will never be forgotten.
My heart grows bigger every day for you.

— D. S. T.

Text copyright © 2019 by Brett Blumenthal and Danielle Shea Tan.
All rights reserved. No part of this book may be reproduced in any form
without written permission from the publisher.

Library of Congress Cataloging-in-Publication Data:
Names: Blumenthal, Brett, author. | Tan, Danielle Shea, author.
Title: 52 small changes for the family / Brett Blumenthal and Danielle Shea Tan.
Other titles: Fifty two small changes for the family
Description: San Francisco : Chronicle Books, [2019] | Includes index.
Identifiers: LCCN 2018011986 | ISBN 9781452169583 (pbk. : alk. paper)
Subjects: LCSH: Families—Health and hygiene.
Classification: LCC RA777.7 .B58 2019 | DDC 613—dc23 LC record available at
https://lccn.loc.gov/2018011986

Manufactured in China.

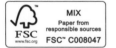

Design by Anne Kenady Smith

Typesetting by Howie Severson

10 9 8 7 6 5 4 3 2

Chronicle books and gifts are available at special quantity discounts to corporations, professional associations, literacy programs, and other organizations. For details and discount information, please contact our premiums
department at corporatesales@chroniclebooks.com or at 1-800-759-0190.

Chronicle Books LLC
680 Second Street
San Francisco, California 94107
www.chroniclebooks.com

CONTENTS

INTRODUCTION

IN OUR COMBINED thirty-plus years in the wellness industry, time and time again we've seen the proof—small changes work. It makes sense: small changes are more realistic and less overwhelming, and they provide us with a quicker sense of accomplishment. Regardless of the change a person wants to make, three things remain true: any major change actually requires many smaller changes; taking an all-or-nothing or extreme approach doesn't work; and small changes that we can manage and master feed our desire to succeed.

Research shows that in order for people to make lasting change or adopt new habits, they must dedicate time to the process. In a study conducted by University College London psychologist Phillippa Lally, individuals who tried to learn new habits, such as eating fruit on a daily basis, took an average of sixty-six days before the behavior had become automatic.[1] In other words, it took subjects an average of nine and a half weeks to make lasting and permanent change. Studies also show when we make small changes over time, we are more likely to be successful than if we try to make large changes all at once.[2] This philosophy was the basis for Brett's first two books in the 52 Small Changes series: 52 Small Changes: One Year to a Happier, Healthier You and 52 Small Changes for the Mind.

After giving birth to our sons, and speaking with other parents with children of various ages, it became all too clear to us that many parents are eager to raise happy, healthy children and are looking for guidance on how to do so. Raising a healthy, balanced, and resilient family may be a common goal, but we've both found that parents struggle with where to begin and what to focus on to best support a child.[3] So it seemed like a natural collaboration to tackle this topic in the 52 Small Changes series, which was originally started by Brett only a few years ago.

52 *Small Changes for the Family* uses the approach of making small changes over the course of a year and applies it specifically to the family unit. It provides parents and caregivers with a detailed guide for improving the health and happiness of their children. Each week for 52 weeks, you are prescribed one habit to incorporate into your family's life, ultimately leading to significant change by the end of the year. Prescribed changes are holistic, addressing multiple areas critical for helping you and your children develop a foundation for optimal health and well-being:

Sharp mind Changes to support healthy cognitive development and intellectual curiosity

Healthy spirit Changes needed for emotional balance, inner personal strength, and emotional intelligence

Resilient body Changes required for a strong body and immune system, including nutrition, physical activity, and overall health changes

Deep connections Changes to develop interpersonal skills for development of strong relationships and community.

Over the course of the next 52 weeks, we hope you and your family find the changes to be fun and relatively easy to implement. But even more important, we hope you all enjoy the process together and that the journey brings you closer together as a family.

Brett Blumenthal
Danielle Shea Tan

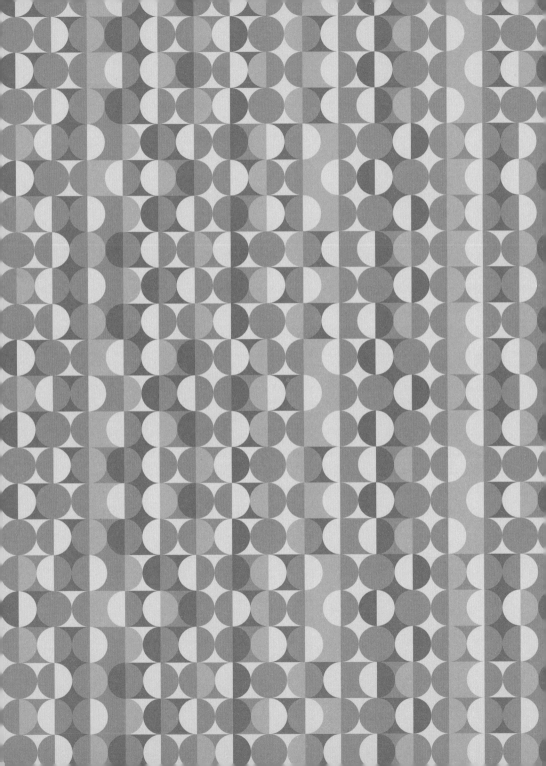

THE PROGRAM

HOW IT WORKS

THE 52 SMALL CHANGES FOR THE FAMILY program is designed to encourage small yet meaningful changes that will ultimately lead you and your family to enjoy a happier, healthier lifestyle. The idea is simple: make one small change per week for 52 weeks, and at the end of the year, you and your children will benefit from increased mental clarity, curiosity, and focus; better emotional balance and strength; improved physical health; and deeper connections with friends and family and, most important, with one another. This book is designed with two things in mind:

1. Giving you and your family a year to make changes enables you to slowly integrate them over time, so they are more likely to stick for the long term.

2. Although there are countless changes you can make, the changes presented in this book are small enough that they won't be overwhelming, yet will have significant impact.

Each change comes with an explanation as to why the change is important, as well as a "Path to Change," which provides tips and recommendations to help you successfully implement the change. With each week's success, you and your family will be inspired to move to the next week's change, so that, within a year, you'll have mastered all 52 changes.

To best support you in your journey to a healthier, happier family, we've supplied tools, worksheets, and other resources in Part III; we highly recommend you use these to stay motivated and on track throughout the program.

A HOLISTIC APPROACH

The program outlined in 52 *Small Changes for the Family* takes an integrated approach. At the beginning of each week's chapter, you'll see an icon signifying which of the four areas the change addresses. The changes have been organized so all areas are addressed throughout the 52 weeks, instead of one at a time. This will keep you engaged, interested, and motivated, and allow you to comprehensively make progress. The icons are as follows:

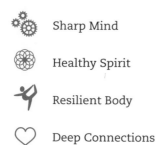

Sharp Mind

Healthy Spirit

Resilient Body

Deep Connections

Every twelve weeks, you'll see the "Quarterly Changes Checklist," which lists the changes you've made up until that point so you can keep track of your progress and be sure to keep integrating the changes into your lifestyle.

LIFE AFTER THE 52 WEEKS

Once you and your family complete the 52-week program, the hope is you'll have increased mental clarity, curiosity, and focus; greater emotional balance and strength; improved physical health; and deeper connections with friends, family, and one another than you do today.

Consistently maintaining all 52 changes, however, may not always be seamless and easy. There may be times when it's a bit challenging or

A HAPPIER, HEALTHIER LIFESTYLE

HERE ARE SOME of the biggest benefits you and your family can look forward to:

+ STRONGER FAMILY CONNECTIONS. By going through this process together as a family, you'll grow together in new ways, developing stronger and deeper connections with one another.

+ A FULLER, MORE REWARDING LIFE. Each member of your family will have more energy, strength, and mental stability, which will allow all of you—particularly your children—to thrive and perform at your best, and your family to enjoy life to the fullest and to feel great in all aspects of life.

+ IMPROVED OUTLOOK. Both you and your children will have a happier, more positive outlook, which will extend into your personal relationships, work, school, extracurricular activities, and other areas of your life.

+ GROWING PAINS AND AGING. Living a healthy lifestyle means making healthy choices, staying active, and feeling energetic, at every age. As a result, children will experience fewer growing pains, and as parents, you'll be able to keep up with your children more easily and feel younger, longer.

+ GREATER SELF-ESTEEM. Taking care of yourselves allows you to feel good both physically and mentally. This directly results in a boost to self-esteem and self-confidence.

+ NATURAL PREVENTION. Taking a proactive approach to living healthy today will prevent the need to be reactive tomorrow. You will ward off common, everyday sickness, as well as prevent your family from developing diseases such as diabetes, cancer, and heart disease.

+ INCREASED CONTROL OF YOUR LIFE. When you and your family are confronted with challenges, you will be better prepared, both physically and mentally, to take them on and make the best of the situation. Children will feel less overwhelmed when presented with life's disappointments and will be able to cope more productively and effectively.

+ RAISED AWARENESS. Through this process, you and your children will become highly aware of the choices you make, which will enable you to listen to your bodies and minds to know what is needed to feel best.

your schedule and your family's make it difficult. Life happens, so be sure not to let slipups discourage you. Life is a constant balancing act and requires us to make sacrifices. When you aren't on top of everything, remember: tomorrow is a new day. Let yourself and your family approach each day with new motivation and resolve. In the end, integrating the prescribed changes *most* of the time is what's most important for you and your children.

Revisit 52 *Small Changes for the Family* often, as it will always provide you with the basis for living a happy, healthy life. And consider making it a yearly project: when one year is completed, return to Week 1 and challenge your family to delve deeper into each of the changes!

GO YOUR OWN WAY

Although we've designed 52 *Small Changes for the Family* to be followed over the course of a year and with a certain progression, it is ultimately your and your family's own personal journey. Use this program in whatever way works best for you. That said, we highly recommend you take at least a week to integrate a small change before moving on to a new one. If one change is really easy or you are already incorporating it into your lifestyle, however, feel free to move forward with a different change.

Additionally, if you don't want to use this book sequentially but prefer to go out of order, that is fine, too. We would emphasize, however, that (1) you take your time so the changes you make stick, and (2) no matter what timeline you use, be sure to incorporate all 52 changes into your and your family's life, as they are meant to work together in concert.

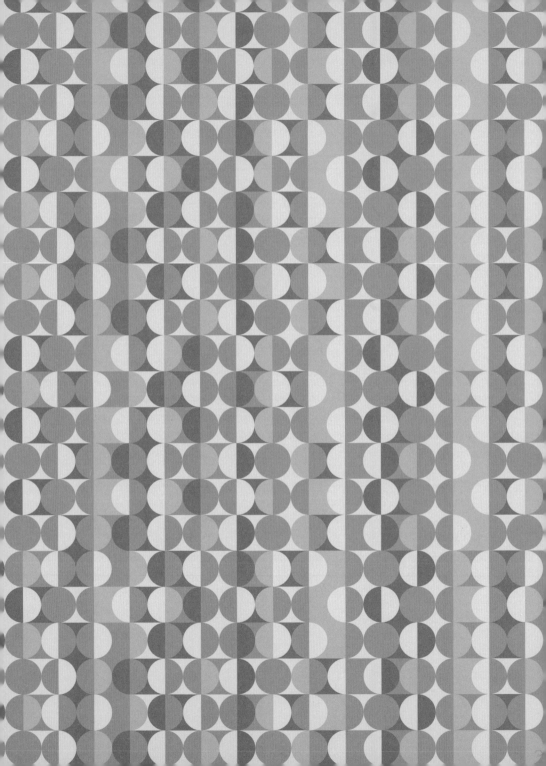

PART II

52 WEEKS OF HABITS

TICKLE YOUR FUNNY BONE

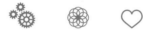

A good laugh heals a lot of hurts.
—Madeleine L'Engle

THOUGH IT MAY seem trite to encourage laughter, given all of the responsibilities of parenting, we all could benefit from more humor. Let's face it—parenting is a tough job. But laughter allows us to enjoy both the good and bad moments, keeps us healthy, and helps maintain our sanity.

Laughter can be the perfect antidote to an otherwise stressful situation. What else can you do but laugh when you lock your family out of the house or step in dog poop? When we laugh, especially with others, our brains release endorphins—neurochemicals that boost our moods, induce calmness, and reduce feelings of pain.[1,2] Endorphins have been known to produce similar effects on the mind as mood-altering drugs such as morphine. Since laughter activates endorphin production, it can also lower blood pressure and heart rate.

In fact, research shows laughter protects the heart and improves vascular function by decreasing arterial stiffness and lowering cortisol, a stress hormone.[3,4] A large study of over twenty thousand Japanese men and women aged sixty-five and older found that people who never or almost never laugh are 121 percent more likely to have cardiovascular disease and 160 percent more likely to have a stroke than those who reported laughing every day.[5]

If that isn't enough to convince you that laughter is the best medicine, consider that laughter boosts your immune system, too.[6,7] Studies show it stimulates the production of natural killer cells, a type of white blood cell that limits the spread of infection and controls tumor growth. Further, research shows people with a strong sense of humor are much less likely to die from cardiovascular disease or infection than their more serious peers.[8]

Beyond health, laughter brings people closer together and has been shown to enhance bonds and relationships.[9] Enjoying laughter can bring more joy and happiness into your family dynamic and provide your children with a coping mechanism that can get them through life's ups and downs. Further, married couples that engage in humor can experience more intimacy, a more positive mindset, and greater satisfaction in their relationships.[10]

DID YOU KNOW?

According to humor and laughter expert Dr. Rod Martin, a person's sense of humor can be attributed to both genetics and environmental factors.[11] If laughter doesn't come easily to you, you can modify your sense of humor to some degree with concerted focus on activities that provide amusement.

THE CHANGE
FIND WAYS TO LAUGH EVERY DAY.

PATH TO CHANGE   Everyone could use a little more laughter. Use the following tips to boost laughter in your family's life:

LAUGH AT YOURSELF   Chuckling when you leave your coffee mug on your car roof or wear slippers to work can defuse an otherwise terrible morning. People who laugh at themselves are certainly fun to be around when the going gets rough, and they also tend to be more cheery and easygoing, and less hampered by failure or change.

According to laughter expert Dr. Rod Martin, self-deprecating humor, or not taking yourself too seriously, leads to more positive experiences in life, whereas self-defeating humor, or disparaging yourself to be accepted by others, does the opposite by bringing on a negative mindset. Keep it light—laugh at your mistakes and embrace your quirks.

TELL JOKES   You don't have to be Jerry Seinfeld to share a good joke; you just need a good joke book. Get your family involved in finding books of jokes that make you all laugh. Preschool children will love learning age-appropriate jokes to share with their friends, while older children will appreciate the lightness of a joke-telling home life.

SEEK HUMOR IN EVERYDAY LIFE   Take cues from the "That's Silly" picture puzzle in the *High Five* magazine for kids, and find things in real life that make your family crack up. Stop to laugh at the dog in the stroller or the mustache on the grill of an SUV. When encouraged, children can find silliness in just about anything.

DRESS UP PLAY   Playing pretend isn't just for toddlers; children and adults of all ages can enjoy a good costume party. Let your younger children create a superhero costume for you or—even funnier—try to wear *their* tiny costumes. Get older children involved by cohosting a costume party with a fun theme, like Sweating to the Oldies or Best of the '80s. You don't have to wait for Halloween; just grab a bunch of silly hats, wigs, and accessories, and start snapping photos—every family member will be giggling in no time.

LAUGHTER AND YOGA: A PERFECT COMBINATION

Laughter yoga is a practice, developed by Dr. Madan Kataria, which intentionally stimulates laughter among participants through making sounds such as rapid "ha-has" and "ho-hos." The yoga practice includes physical movement with a lot of added laughter that may start out sounding fake . . . but eventually brings an eruption of joy to the room. Find a class online or near you at www.laughteryoga.org.

BE SILLY   Find your silly side. Try singing silly songs or making silly faces. Your teens may roll their eyes at your antics, but even middle-school children can laugh aloud at silly games. For younger children, change words to their favorite songs or rhymes to make them sound funny. For older children, add silly games like *Pie Face!* or *Say Anything* to family game night.

READ FUNNY BOOKS   Besides joke books, there are loads of funny books to enjoy. An oldie but goodie is Mad Libs, which allows players to create funny stories with fill-in blanks. Ask librarians for recommendations on age-appropriate humorous books for your children and funny books you can enjoy together. And don't forget to try a humorous book for your own reading pleasure.

MAKE FUNNY MOMENTS VISIBLE   Although smartphones make capturing real-life silly moments easy, the photos often get buried. Print silly pictures to make them visible so you can recall laughable memories at your desk, in the kitchen, or when driving. Use photo apps such as Chatbooks (www.chatbooks.com) or Snapfish (www.snapfish.com), which link directly to your phone, so you can print photos at home or turn them into treasured memory books.

SLEEP SOUNDLY

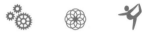

> It is a common experience that a problem difficult at night is resolved in the morning after the committee of sleep has worked on it.
> —JOHN STEINBECK

QUALITY SLEEP IS critical to your family's health and longevity. During sleep, the immune system heals and rejuvenates your body. The brain converts new information into memory and forms new neural connections that enhance cognitive function, such as problem-solving and creativity. Emotional processing that regulates mood, behavior, and emotions also occurs during nighttime sleep. Though sleep was once thought to be an inactive time for the brain, scientists have since discovered the brain may be more active while we sleep than when we are awake.[1]

DID YOU KNOW?
Sleep deprivation for just one night lowers immune response and raises inflammatory markers that persist even after you get another full night's sleep. Chronic inflammation is believed to be the root cause of many common diseases.[2]

Despite the importance of high-quality sleep, many parents and children are sleep deprived. A 2013 Gallup poll found parents of children under eighteen are one of the most sleep-deprived populations, with only 52 percent indicating they get at least seven hours of sleep nightly, the minimum recommendation.[3] Further, the American Academy of Pediatrics (AAP) refers to teen sleep deprivation as an epidemic. Rightly so, as an analysis of over 270,000 teens found that less than two-thirds of sixteen- to seventeen-year-olds and one-third of fourteen- to fifteen-year-olds report getting the nine hours of sleep each night recommended.[4]

As parents, we can all attest to the noticeable differences in joy and coping skills between a well-rested child and a sleep-deprived one. The effect of chronic sleep deprivation on family health and happiness, however, goes beyond a little whining. Research shows inadequate sleep not only causes sleepiness in children but also produces issues with attention, impulse control, behavioral regulation, and academic performance.[5] Children with sleep problems are also more likely to develop anxiety and depression in the future.[6,7,8,9]

Sleep deprivation impedes the mind's ability to manage emotions and make rational decisions. In fact, teens with poor sleep engage in more risky behaviors, including unprotected sexual intercourse, violence, and the use of tobacco, alcohol, marijuana, or illegal drugs.[10] Sleep deprivation also affects physical health and has been associated with weight gain, a weak metabolism, and compromised immune function. These physiological consequences are factors that link poor-quality sleep or lack of sleep to many medical conditions including high blood pressure, heart attack, heart failure, and stroke.[11] It turns out sleep is just as important to good physical health as exercise and nutrition.

When it comes to making sleep a priority, parents have the most influential position. Parental sleep behaviors and attitudes about the importance of sleep are noticeable to children and impact their ability to practice good sleep habits and achieve healthy sleep. For example, a recent study found parental sleep duration and the confidence a parent feels in his or her ability to help children get quality sleep directly affects children's sleep duration.[12] Taking steps to improve your own sleep patterns is just as important as teaching children how to experience high-quality sleep.

THE CHANGE
PRIORITIZE HEALTHY SLEEP.

PATH TO CHANGE   Getting quality sleep takes effort, especially as we age. Use the following evidence-informed suggestions to support your family in developing healthy sleep behaviors that last a lifetime:

ESTABLISH SLEEP RULES   Parents who prioritize sleep and set limits around sleep/wake times for the entire family will demonstrate the importance of sleep. Sleep experts suggest adult and adolescent sleep should ideally commence between 8 p.m. and midnight and continue for seven to nine hours.[13] A younger child's ideal bedtime is generally between 6:30 and 8:30 p.m. Setting parameters for "lights out" times that align with these suggested time frames increases the likelihood that all family members will get quality sleep. While older children can easily follow sleep limits, parents of younger children may need to get creative. For instance, consider purchasing alarm clocks designed with "time to wake" and "time to sleep" color patterns, pictures, and/or sounds to designate sleep and wake times.

SLEEP RECOMMENDATIONS BY AGE[14]

AGE	RECOMMENDED SLEEP DURATION IN EACH 24-HOUR PERIOD	DANGEROUS SLEEP DURATION IN EACH 24-HOUR PERIOD
0 to 3 months	14 to 17 hours	<11 hours, >19 hours
4 to 11 months	12 to 15 hours	<10 hours, >18 hours
1 to 2 years	11 to 14 hours	<9 hours, >16 hours
3 to 5 years	10 to 13 hours	<8 hours, >14 hours
6 to 13 years	9 to 11 hours	<7 hours, >12 hours
14 to 17 years	8 to 10 hours	<7 hours, >11 hours
18 to 25 years	7 to 9 hours	<6 hours, >11 hours
26 to 64 years	7 to 9 hours	<6 hours, >10 hours
>65 years	7 to 8 hours	<5 hours, >9 hours

CREATE A SLEEP-INDUCING ENVIRONMENT The right environment makes all the difference when it comes to achieving quality sleep.

Darkness Sunlight and artificial light impede production of melatonin, the hormone responsible for sleep. While some adults may enjoy waking up to natural light, children are more sensitive to light during sleep. Use light-blocking shades or curtains to help children sleep as long as needed (and if you are light-sensitive, use them yourself). When young children request nightlights, choose a warm color and place the light out of direct line of sight.

Temperature During sleep, we are less able to regulate body temperature, so room temperature is important for quality sleep. Studies show keeping bedroom temperatures on the cooler side, optimally between 60°F (15°C) and 68°F (20°C), is best.[15] Be sure children have plenty of layered bedding to keep them warm or cool. For winter months or drafty homes, keep young children warm with heavier pajamas or wearable blankets.

Noise/white noise For light sleepers, even the quietest noises, such as a creaky stair, can cause sleep disturbances. Use a white noise machine to help children and adults sleep through the normal noises of a busy household. But be mindful of the volume of these machines, as white noise machines that are too loud may impact hearing.

Electromagnetic fields All objects, even humans, contain electrical charges and produce a physical field referred to as an EMF. Electrical devices produce stronger EMFs; power transmission lines produce one of the strongest forms of EMF. Some studies show EMF exposure can impact health, including sleep quality. To reduce EMF exposure, turn off your home's wireless network at night, remove all electronic devices from the bedrooms, and consider purchasing an EMF protection unit.

Nighttime clothing Choose materials best suited to each family member. For family members who sleep hot, choose bedding made from bamboo fibers, which naturally wick away moisture from the body. And those who tend to get cold, choose flannel, a breathable material made from wool or cotton. In warmer seasons, plain cotton is a good option since it is both breathable and comfortable.

Establish nighttime routines   Nighttime routines help children wind down from the day and prepare for sleep. Routines can include preparing for the next day, bathing, reading, meditating, gentle massage, journaling, and more. Make nighttime routines especially relaxing by dimming all lights, speaking in quiet voices, and moving slowly from task to task.

AVOID SLEEP DISRUPTORS   Although many sleep disruptors may not be noticeable during the night, they can still impact your sleep, making you feel less rested in the morning or groggy throughout the day.

Missing naps   Naps for young children are just as important as nighttime sleep. Infants and children up to age thirty months who do not nap are not getting adequate sleep for their age. And some children will need naps even through age five. Find support in the "Get Help for Common Sleep Challenges" section at the end this chapter.

Napping too late   Naps too close to bedtime can disrupt sleep patterns. It should take no longer than twenty to thirty minutes for children and adults to fall asleep. If young children take more than twenty minutes to fall asleep, consider modifying their nap schedule and bedtime routines to ensure they are ready for bed at the designated time.

Blue light   Blue light wavelengths are most powerful in suppressing the production of melatonin. Blue light is emitted by most electronic devices, including televisions, tablets, smartphones, computers, and alarm clocks. Remove blue light sources from bedrooms to minimize the impact.

Alcohol   Although alcohol seemingly relaxes, it has been shown to cause sleep disruption. Finish drinking alcohol at least three hours before bedtime to minimize disruptions.

Caffeine after 2 p.m.   Scientists have found genetic differences in how caffeine affects individuals—some people clear caffeine from the bloodstream more quickly than others.[16] For most people, caffeine (found in chocolate, coffee, and tea) acts as a stimulant and can alter circadian rhythms, which can keep us up and disrupt our natural sleep/wake cycle.

NATURAL SLEEP PROMOTERS

MANY NATURAL REMEDIES are associated with improvements in sleep. Try the following suggestions to maintain healthy sleep.

+ **LAVENDER ESSENTIAL OIL:** This fragrance has physiological properties that promote relaxation and sleep. See Week 17, Smell the Aroma to incorporate essential oils into a nighttime routine.

+ **EPSOM SALT BATH:** The magnesium in Epsom salt—a mineral needed for proper muscle relaxation—promotes relaxation and soothes sore muscles. Salt baths are not recommended for children under age 5.

+ **EXERCISE:** Regular daily exercise promotes healthy sleep by shortening the time it takes to fall asleep and lengthening the duration of sound sleep.[17] And exercise before bedtime has been associated with better sleep patterns.[18]

+ **RESTORATIVE YOGA:** A style of yoga focusing on full body relaxation has been shown to improve insomnia in cancer patients.[19]

+ **MEDITATION:** A regular meditation practice can lower stress, improve heart health, and support healthy sleep. Use a meditation phone app suitable for adults and/or children, or download meditation guides for screen-free listening.

+ **TUI NA MASSAGE OR GENTLE MASSAGE:** This ancient form of Chinese massage uses gentle stimulation of specific acupressure points to achieve desired results. Find guided instructional videos from leading pediatric acupuncturist Robin Green, L.Ac. MTCM on her website (www.kidsloveacupuncture.com) or on YouTube.

+ **HOMEOPATHIC REMEDIES:** Developed in the nineteenth century by Dr. Samuel Christian Hahnemann, a German physician, homeopathy is a type of medicine that uses highly diluted substances to treat common ailments. Try sleep formulas from Hyland's, Ollois, and Dr. King's, or consider seeing a classic homeopath who develops customized formulas.

Large meals within three hours of bedtime Eating a large meal too close to bedtime results in a rapid drop in blood sugar during sleep. This raises cortisol, the stress hormone, while inhibiting melatonin release. Going to bed hungry will also cause sleep disruption. If family members eat dinner early, they may need a snack after dinner to achieve quality sleep. Serve small, well-balanced snacks that incorporate some healthy fats, such as apples and nut butter, or carrots and hummus.

Pharmacological sleep aids Many prescribed sleep aids are addictive and produce many unwanted side effects. Weaning from sleep aids, however, requires guidance from a supportive physician or medical practitioner. Many of the natural remedies included in this section can support healthy sleep without unwanted side effects.

Medications Medications prescribed for other health conditions can disrupt sleep patterns. If you are on any medications and are experiencing difficulties getting good-quality sleep, speak with your doctor to see if any of your medications might be to blame.

Smoking Many smokers sleep very lightly and often wake up in the middle of the night or early in the morning due to nicotine withdrawal. Ideally, no one in your family smokes. If any of you do, you can improve sleep and overall health and boost longevity by quitting using methods including hypnosis or nicotine replacement therapy.

GET HELP FOR COMMON SLEEP CHALLENGES   If you and your child struggle with getting quality sleep, talking to sleep consultants trained to help families solve normal sleep challenges can be very helpful. Find a sleep consultant whose sleep philosophy and approach aligns with your values and comfort level. Sleep apnea, heavy snoring, and breathing issues can cause sleep disorders. If you feel someone in your family is suffering from chronic sleep deprivation, seek out the help of a sleep specialist or speak to your primary care physician. Also, several nationally recognized sleep experts have written quality books to guide parents through even the most difficult sleep challenges.

HYDRATE HEALTHFULLY

If there is magic on this planet, it is contained in water.
—Loren Eiseley

WATER IS VITAL to proper body function and is often considered the fourth macronutrient by nutritionists, along with protein, fat, and carbohydrates. Every cell in the body relies on pure water for metabolic processes. In fact, 60 percent of an adult's body weight and 70 percent of an infant's weight is made up of water.[1] Losing just 1 to 2 percent of body weight from dehydration impacts emotional balance, cognitive function, and physical performance.[2] And, though we may not realize it, we are constantly losing water throughout the day through sweat, urine, feces, and exhalation.

PREVENTION THROUGH HYDRATION

Despite water's importance, almost seventy-four thousand children (ages one to eighteen) are admitted to the hospital each year for dehydration.[3] And according to a study published in *Hospital Pediatrics*, at least 45 percent of these hospital stays are preventable. The key is educating families on daily water intake recommendations and offering children more clear fluids throughout the day. Further, many medical and nutrition experts feel that most Americans are not drinking nearly enough water for optimal health. In fact, a 2007 study by the Centers for Disease Control (CDC) found 43 percent of Americans reported drinking less than four cups of water daily, or less than half of the average recommended daily intake.[4]

Water maintains proper blood volume, which supports healthy blood pressure and effective circulation. It also carries oxygen to the skin and lungs, keeping them supple and lubricated so they can effectively defend against infection. The kidneys and colon need water to flush toxins, aid digestion, and ease elimination. In fact, drinking more water is the first therapy recommended to children and adults experiencing constipation. Without adequate water, your family may experience fatigue, reduced mental clarity, impaired short- and long-term memory, inability to pay attention, trouble regulating body temperature, constipation, and urinary tract issues.

Just as parents directly influence their children's eating habits, they also influence their drinking habits. For example, a study found children and adults from the same family tend to consume similar calories from sweetened beverages every day—an indication that children drink what their parents drink.[5] Put simply, when parents prioritize water, children will, too.

THE CHANGE
PRIORITIZE WATER FOR DRINKING.

PATH TO CHANGE   Keep your family properly hydrated to maximize energy, metabolism, and brain function and realize improved health. Use the following tips to get started:

KNOW YOUR FAMILY'S NEEDS   Daily water requirements vary by individual and environmental factors including height, weight, physical activity, air temperature, and humidity. Consider the following guidelines when helping your family stay hydrated.

Needs There are several common methods for estimating daily water requirements, but most nutritionists use weight as a general measure for adults. Drink the amount of water in ounces that equals your weight in pounds, divided by two. For example, an adult who weighs 160 pounds should aim to drink 80 ounces or ten 8-ounce cups of water per day. Water requirements for children vary by age as follows:

DAILY DRINKING WATER REQUIREMENTS FOR CHILDREN[6]

AGE	AVERAGE 8-OUNCE CUPS PER DAY
4 to 8 years	5
9 to 13 years (girls)	7
9 to 13 years (boys)	8
14 to 18 years (girls)	8
14 to 18 years (boys)	11

Exercise It is important to hydrate during exercise to avoid muscle cramping and dehydration. Drink when you are thirsty, of course, and if any family member does not recognize thirst during exercise, encourage drinking some fluids anyway. All physical activity increases fluid loss through sweating, even if sweat is not visible. When engaged in prolonged exercise (over two hours), use electrolyte drinks to properly rehydrate and replenish lost sodium—try unsweetened coconut water, a naturally healthy and delicious electrolyte drink that's appropriate for children ages one and older.

Hot climates Keep all family members hydrated with extra fluids when it's hot. Offer cold beverages, make ice pops with water and fruit, and, for snacks, serve produce with a high water content, such as cucumbers, watermelon, and grapes.

SERVE WATER   Offer water with every meal and snack to ensure that all family members have access to plenty of fluids throughout the day. Make water readily available by keeping a pitcher of cold water in the fridge or placing cups next to the sink so all family members, including younger children, can get a drink.

USE BPA-FREE WATER BOTTLES   You'll naturally encourage water consumption by making sure every family member carries a reusable water bottle. Choose bottles made of stainless steel or glass with a silicone sleeve to avoid unnecessary exposure to chemicals in plastic bottles.

Old plastic bottles Avoid reusing old plastic water bottles from water or other beverages. They are often made of thin plastic that breaks down with time, ultimately leaching chemicals into your water. Older plastic bottles can also harbor bacteria that get stuck in the cracks and scratches caused by wear and tear.

Family-size thermos You can ensure water is available at all times with a family-size thermos (approximately 64 ounces). Bring a water-filled thermos along whenever your family leaves the house. You can use the thermos to refill reusable water bottles or serve water in small stainless steel camping cups.

MAKE IT TASTY   If your family does not enjoy the taste of plain water, try adding chopped fresh produce, such as cucumbers, oranges, strawberries, raspberries, lemons, or limes, to give it a bit of flavor. When all else fails, add a splash of 100 percent fruit juice to water.

EAT YOUR WATER Most fruits and vegetables contain over 80 percent water, another great reason to serve more produce! When kids are eating a healthy, balanced diet they'll typically get 25 percent of their water needs in the form of food. Try serving fruit and/or veggies with every meal and snack for a tasty way to keep them hydrated and healthy.

SERVE LIQUID MEALS OR SNACKS Water is a key ingredient in healthy recipes for homemade smoothies, soups, and even fresh fruit ice pops, which are tasty and fun to eat! Serve smoothies and homemade ice pops for breakfast or snack-time hydration. To ensure that your kids are well hydrated when they aren't with you, purchase a well-insulated thermos so they can bring liquid meals to school or day care.

WATCH OUT FOR DEHYDRATING FLUIDS Pure water is the ideal way to hydrate. Bottled drinks like Vitaminwater, Gatorade, Powerade, and other flavored waters often contain artificial ingredients, preservatives, sugar, and empty calories that are not good for your health. Although drinking 100 percent juice provides some vitamins and minerals, it is also high in sugar and should be consumed in moderation. And some beverages have been shown to dehydrate the body, requiring a person to drink more water. Consider the following information when choosing which beverages to serve your family; you'll need to compensate for diuretic beverages by drinking extra hydrating fluids:

HYDRATION STATUS OF COMMON BEVERAGES

BEVERAGE NAME	HYDRATES (+) / DEHYDRATES (−)	CONSIDERATIONS
Alcohol	−	Alcohol is a diuretic.
Carbonated water	+	Check that it is sodium-free.
Coconut water	+	This all-natural electrolyte drink is a good rehydrater; choose versions without added sugar.

BEVERAGE NAME	HYDRATES (+) / DEHYDRATES (-)	CONSIDERATIONS
Coffee	–	Caffeine is a diuretic.
Diet soda	–	Artificial sweeteners are shown to cause headaches, fatigue, and other symptoms, including developing a distaste for healthy foods that lack extreme sweetness.
Fruit juice (100 percent)	+	Because it's high in sugar, The American Heart Association (AHA) and many nutritionists recommend no more than 8 ounces weekly of beverages sweetened with sugar, including juice.[8]
Milk	+	Traditional cow's milk (or goat's milk) naturally contains some electrolytes. Alternative dairy products such as almond milk can also be hydrating; be sure to choose sugar-free versions.
Plain water	+	This is the best liquid to replenish lost fluids.
Soda	–	It's high in sugar, and caffeinated soda is a diuretic.
Sports drinks	+	These often contain artificial ingredients and sweeteners shown to cause headaches, fatigue, and other symptoms.
Tea (Herbal)	+/-	Black tea has caffeine, a diuretic. Some white and green tea varieties are lower in caffeine and can be used to hydrate.

KNOW THE SIGNS OF DEHYDRATION The symptoms of dehydration can differ by age. For adults, symptoms include extreme thirst, less frequent urination, dark urine, fatigue, confusion, dizziness, and irritability. For infants and children, tears should be produced when crying and a wet diaper should be produced every three hours. Also, check that children's mouths and tongues are properly lubricated. In severe dehydration, children can become listless or have sunken eyes or cheeks, and infants can have a sunken soft spot on the top of the skull.[9]

BE A BOOKWORM

The more that you read, the more things you will know.
The more that you learn, the more places you'll go.

—Dr. Seuss

READING BEDTIME STORIES is an age-old tradition that invokes heart-warming memories for most of us. And since reading has been shown to reduce stress, it is also a perfect way to relax into slumber.[1] Once a child learns to read, this favorite pastime need not end. Children of all ages, including tweens and teens, enjoy being read to, and continue to flourish from the benefits.

With the explosive growth of technology, reading for pleasure may become a thing of the past for older kids. The National Center for Education Statistics indicates the population of teens who read for pleasure daily has dropped from 35 percent to 27 percent among thirteen-year-olds and from 31 percent to 19 percent among seventeen-year-olds.[2] Yet reading is a critical skill that requires repetition and constant practice for continued development and mastery.

Unlike watching television or videos, reading is an active process that develops neural pathways, which makes us smarter. In one study, researchers scanned the brains of children ages three to five as they listened to prerecorded stories. They observed activity in several areas of the left side of the brain, and this activity was higher in children who lived in a more literacy-friendly home.[3] The more you read to your children, provide access to books, and offer literary variety, the more your children's brain neurons will develop, increasing their abilities in comprehension, vocabulary, and language fluency.

Reading, whether done aloud to your child or independently, enhances creativity by allowing a child to personalize the images from a story using his own imagination. Reading also offers children both academic and emotional benefits. One study found that reading to children builds literacy skills more than talking to them. Researchers found vocabulary used in picture books to be more extensive than the five thousand most common English words used in conversation with children.[4] According to research by Thomas Sticht, children have a higher level of listening comprehension than reading comprehension. They need to hear words in context before they can speak them or understand them while reading. So the younger the age at which a child is exposed to more advanced books and words, the higher the child's vocabulary and literacy level.[5]

Parents are the most influential people to develop their children's love and regular practice of reading.[6] Children of all ages enjoy being read aloud to, even older children. According to several studies of middle schoolers, when teachers read aloud to students, a teaching practice that's slowly been on the rise in America, the students' levels of motivation, interest, and engagement in the content was enhanced.[7]

Adopting your own personal reading rituals provides amazing benefits to the health of your brain and mental well-being. No matter your age, reading stimulates creativity, reduces stress, improves focus and concentration, and sharpens your mind as you gain new knowledge and strengthen your language skills.

THE CHANGE
READ TOGETHER.

PATH TO CHANGE   Reading with children is not only beneficial to mental well-being but can bring your family closer together as well. Over 82 percent of children identify parents as the most influential person who inspired them to read.[9] Try the following strategies to make reading a fun priority for every family member:

MAKE READING PART OF YOUR ROUTINE   Integrate reading into your routine so that it becomes a natural part of your day.

Read to sleep   Incorporate reading into bedtime routines. Start bedtime early to give your family plenty of time to enjoy several books together. Though tweens are reading on their own, studies show they still love to be read to by loved ones.[10]

Read to relax   Schedule a regular time to relax and read books together to decompress from the hustle of modern life. Make it a weekly, if not daily, event so your family can benefit on a regular basis.

Read on vacation   Vacations are most beneficial if the schedule allows adults and children to find quiet time. When going on vacation, make it a ritual to choose new books to enjoy during your time away. This includes summer breaks: children who enjoy books throughout the summer will avoid the "summer slide"—the loss of reading comprehension skills when kids aren't in school.

BRING THEM EVERYWHERE   Instead of bringing along toys to keep younger children occupied during errands, tuck a few exciting new books in your bag. Model this behavior so older children get accustomed to bringing their own reading materials, too.

DID YOU KNOW?

Children of all ages love to listen to stories by loved ones. According to a report by Scholastic Books, the frequency of reading aloud dramatically drops with age—59 percent (infant to five years old), 38 percent (six to eight), and 17 percent (nine to eleven)—yet 87 percent of kids ages six to eleven said they loved reading books aloud with parents. Children report enjoying this special time together because it's fun and relaxing, and they can enjoy books too difficult to read by themselves.[11]

VISIT LIBRARIES   Take your family to the local library. Since libraries are filled with books from all time periods, the discoveries are endless! Most libraries have children's areas, so you can let younger kids explore on their own. When your children find books they are excited about, check them out so they can enjoy them at home.

GIVE BOOK GIFTS   For birthdays and holidays, consider giving your children gift certificates to a bookstore. Explore the whole store, as most bookstores are designed to entice and inspire young readers. Check out staff picks, and relax and enjoy the adventure by test-driving a few books in some comfy chairs before making a purchase.

SIGN UP FOR BOOK CLUBS   Book clubs are a great way to motivate young readers and provide them with opportunities to connect with other kids to reflect and discuss books of interest. Encourage your children to join a book club or start one of their own.

USE BOOKS TO TEACH LESSONS   Guiding children through stories is an effective education strategy for social and emotional learning. Children can relate to characters in the stories without the complication of parental pressure. You can find stories to support children through everything from potty training to money management. Ask friends, teachers, librarians, or local bookstore staff for recommendations.

HELP CHILDREN FIND BOOKS   Children often lose interest in reading when it becomes difficult to find books they enjoy. Surprisingly, 41 percent of all children and 57 percent of infrequent readers have trouble finding books they enjoy.[12] Ask other parents and librarians for book and series recommendations so you can guide your family in findings books they love.

TRY AUDIOBOOKS   Audiobooks offer adults and children access to thousands of titles through apps available on most devices. Although many parents use audiobooks as a means of reducing screen time, they also help children fall in love with the practice of reading. Children of all ages benefit from audiobooks because listening to stories beyond their reading level can enhance literacy development and expand vocabulary. For added benefit, the child can follow along with the book on paper.

GO DIGITAL   Personal electronic devices and eReaders provide access to a vast number of titles that bookstores and libraries may not have. If your older children are glued to their devices, help them find digital books that spark their interest. If you're heading off on a trip, choose digital books to make it easier (and lighter) to bring books for the whole family to enjoy.

EXPERIENCE LIVE STORYTELLING   Older children and adults can enjoy live and recorded performances of stories told by the authors themselves. The Moth, a nonprofit organization whose mission is to promote the art and craft of storytelling, hosts podcasts and runs live storytelling events in most metropolitan areas.

MINIMIZE AND ORGANIZE

The objective of cleaning is not just to clean, but to feel happiness living within that environment.

—MARIE KONDO

AS CHILDREN ENTER different ages and stages of life, families tend to accumulate more and more stuff. This clutter collects on counters, in the entryway, on the coffee table, under the bathroom sink, and, of course, in closets. Though it may seem like a minor concern in the grand scheme of life, clutter and disorder take a toll on your family's health.

Studies show physical clutter competes for our attention more than we realize, wearing us down and increasing cortisol (stress hormone) levels.[1,2] Children are especially vulnerable to the effects of disorder and disarray in their physical environment. One study found that household chaos, a term that includes household clutter and disorder, was associated with lower health outcomes for children.[3] And it's no wonder! "Dust mites, pet dander and mold lurk in physical possessions, which can trigger allergic reactions, decrease air quality and increase potential asthma problems," says Dr. Uma Gavani, an allergy and asthma specialist.[4]

Reducing clutter and unnecessary items in your home creates more physical space for your family to enjoy while freeing up mental space for improved focus, productivity, and learning. Plus, the whole family will spend less time straightening up, cleaning, and searching for lost items.

DID YOU KNOW?

Household disorder can affect a child's reading ability. Researchers from Columbia University conducted a study of 455 families with children in kindergarten or first grade. The study found the degree of household order was strongly associated with three early reading skills, including expressive vocabulary. The more disordered the home, the lower the children's reading capabilities.[5]

THE CHANGE
MINIMIZE CLUTTER, WHILE ORGANIZING YOUR SPACE.

PATH TO CHANGE   Streamlining your home will clear mental and physical space for your family to experience more joy, mental clarity, and productivity. Start tackling clutter with these effective techniques:

DEVISE A PLAN   Create a plan outlining goals for each week or month, and a strategy for making decisions about items. Maintain flexibility in your plan so you can incorporate ideas from your children, too.

Start small Have everyone start with an area that's easy to tackle. Quick wins like cleaning under the bathroom sink or in the entryway closet can uplift your spirit, provide a sense of accomplishment, and inspire you to forge ahead. As small projects are completed, you can join together to tackle bigger areas and rooms in your home.

MAKE IT ROUTINE   Removing clutter is often an extra project added to the bottom of your never-ending to-do list. When you have children, clutter can miraculously reappear in a single evening. Create a weekly clutter management challenge where all family members find clothes or toys to donate and papers to recycle. Dedicate a basket or bin for donations and give it a permanent location in the house. Finally, make it routine by performing it at the same day and time each week.

FIND A HOME FOR EVERYTHING   When items have a home, children of all ages can participate in cleanup. Choose places that mesh with your typical routine. For instance, if receipts collect on the counter, tuck a small expandable folder into the closest cabinet. Have all members of the family choose homes for relevant items so all of you can stay on top of clutter.

DON'T FORGET THE FRIDGE   Typically packed with everything from artwork and menus to bills and permission slips, the fridge, according to UCLA CLEF researchers, is a symbolic representation of clutter that dominates the rest of the house.[6] When your fridge is cluttered it cues the family to allow clutter around the rest of the house, too. Tackle the fridge by first tossing menus, school schedules, and other printed information that can be found online. Next, throw out magnets that don't work and file away old receipts and lingering papers. Use a photo album or envelope for old photos.

ONE IN, ONE OUT   Think about the number of worn towels, ratty stuffed animals, and holey socks taking up space in your home. Adopting the "one in, one out" approach will keep these items to a minimum. Every time a new item enters the house, an older version is decommissioned. Let family members each choose one or two items to be exempt from this rule, such as LEGOs, books, chargers for electronics, jewelry, or collectibles. It's ruthless, but this tactic works wonders for families!

BEFRIEND THE SUN

I will be the gladdest thing under the sun! I will touch
a hundred flowers and not pick one.

—EDNA ST. VINCENT MILLAY

YOU KNOW IT all too well: the sunscreen application wrestling match.
Kids hate it, and parents despise it even more. Though it's become an
obligatory parenting routine, it may be the culprit in a national vitamin
deficiency. Our culture lives in fear of the sun—and rightfully so, since
repetitive sunburns can lead to skin cancer. Despite this challenge, the
most efficient way for the body to synthesize adequate vitamin D is
through sun exposure on bare skin.

Vitamin D is critical for healthy bone development—an important
consideration for children, since peak bone mass is achieved before age
thirty. Without vitamin D, calcium cannot be absorbed. Over five hundred
genes in the body depend on vitamin D, making it instrumental to many
critical biological processes, including the regulation of blood pressure,
blood sugar, and the immune system. Evidence suggests that vitamin D
can also reduce asthma attacks, and it's being researched for its efficacy in reducing the risk of airway infections. Further, studies suggest
symptoms of depression and seasonal affective disorder may be due to
insufficient vitamin D.[1,2]

Most people, including many physicians, do not understand that vitamin D deficiency is associated with increased risk and severity of a host of conditions, including type 1 diabetes, multiple sclerosis, colorectal cancer, breast cancer, rheumatoid arthritis, and lupus.[3] The good news: boosting your family's vitamin D level is a prevention strategy you can control!

The minimum healthy blood level of vitamin D tends to be debated within the medical community. Many respected medical doctors and institutions believe the Recommended Dietary Allowance (RDA) for vitamin D is far too low for optimal health. For example, one study by the U.S. National Heart, Lung and Blood Institute found that, when applying the Canadian Pediatric Society's recommendations for optimal vitamin D levels, two out of three American children (ages one to eleven) are vitamin D deficient.[4] Regardless of the debate, your family can benefit from added vitamin D through safe sun exposure or high-quality supplementation. And when it comes to getting vitamin D through sun exposure, you don't have to worry about getting too much vitamin D. The skin has a built-in mechanism to halt vitamin D production when adequate levels are reached.[5]

DAILY INTAKE RECOMMENDATIONS BY SOURCE[6,7,8,9]

ORGANIZATION	ADULT	PREGNANT/ LACTATING MOTHER	CHILDREN	INFANTS
Vitamin D Council	5,000 IU/ day	4,000 to 6,000 IU/day	1,000 IU/day per 25 lbs. of weight	1,000 IU/ day
The Endocrine Society	1,500 to 2,000 IU/ day	1,500 to 2,000 IU/day	600 to 1,000 IU/ day	400 to 1,000 IU/ day
Institute of Medicine's Food and Nutrition Board	600 to 800 IU/ day	600 IU/day	600 IU/day	400 IU/day

THE CHANGE
GET HEALTHY SUN EXPOSURE.

PATH TO CHANGE Use the following strategies to naturally and safely increase your family's vitamin D levels through healthy sun exposure:

A LITTLE GOES A LONG WAY Being safe in the sun does not require your family to avoid exposure to it completely. Let your family get direct exposure without sunscreen for a short time to allow vitamin D synthesis to occur. Fair-skinned family members may need only a few minutes, whereas dark-skinned family members may require much more time. According to the Vitamin D Council, adequate vitamin D is synthesized in half the time it takes for skin to turn pink before it burns.[11] Expose as much skin as possible to shorten the time needed.

AVOID PEAK SUN Peak sun, typically noontime, is when the sun is strongest and highest in the sky in your area. Vitamin D synthesis does not require direct exposure during peak sun. In fact, since the sun is strongest during this time and more likely to cause sunburns, it's better for your family to be protected or to avoid it completely.

UNDERSTANDING SUN PROTECTION FACTOR (SPF)

Sunscreens are labeled according to their sun protection factor, or SPF. This is the product's ability to screen out the sun's burning rays (UVB). Generally speaking, if it takes you fifteen minutes to burn, wearing sunscreen with SPF 10 should allow you to be in the sun for 10x that time, a total of 15 x 10 = 150 minutes. Keep in mind that SPF does not encompass the product's ability to protect from UVA rays, which penetrate deeper into skin and are harder to block with sunscreen.[12]

CHOOSING AN SPF   Select a sunblock with an SPF that matches your expected activity level and duration of sun exposure. Products with very high SPF (50+ SPF) are misleading and can be harmful to your health because they lull people to stay in the sun longer. Instead, choose a product with an SPF between 30 and 50 to block at least 97 percent of the UVB rays and act as a reminder to limit sun exposure.

MINERAL VERSUS CHEMICAL SUNSCREENS   In general, look for mineral-based sunblocks that contain zinc oxide or titanium dioxide, which create a physical barrier to protect skin from the sun. Try to avoid those sunscreens that use chemicals, such as oxybenzone, avobenzone, octisalate, octocrylene, homosalate, and octinoxate. See Week 40, Clean Up the Chemicals, to learn more about which chemicals to avoid in sunscreen.

CHOOSING A BRAND   There are a zillion sunscreens on the market. Visit the Environmental Working Group's Skin Deep website (www.ewg.org/skindeep) for the latest recommendations for sunscreens that are less toxic and provide good coverage for your family's needs.

APPLY PROPERLY   Applying sunscreen to squirmy children can be a nightmare. After your family has adequate direct exposure for their vitamin D, apply sunscreen to all parts of the body that risk exposure. The scalp, tops of feet, and ears are often overlooked and can easily burn. Apply liberally to all parts of the body in the same way you would apply lotion. While sprays may seem like an easier option, they can contain dangerous inhalants and can be toxic to the environment. Further, when using sprays, it can be easy to miss important parts of the body.

SUN-PROTECTIVE CLOTHING   To avoid missing spots, consider having children wear sun-protective clothing. Sun shirts and hats with UV protection of UPF 40+ are widely available for adults and children. UPF is the rating system used for clothing and hats and refers to the fabric's ability to protect skin from exposure to ultraviolet light. Fabric with a UPF rating of 40+ provides excellent protection as it allows only 2.5% of the UV radiation to reach the protected skin. Everyone can wear these in and out of the water for complete protection from sun exposure. Washing and extensive wear can affect UPF rating, so check the manufacturer's label for instructions on laundering and wear. Also, don't overlook eye protection, and consider sunglasses with UV protection for both you and your children.

SUPPLEMENT IN THE WINTER   Unless your family lives as far south as Miami, Florida, their skin cannot make vitamin D from sun exposure between the months of November and March. During these winter months, the sun and its UVB rays are too far from the Northern Hemisphere. Especially in winter, it's best to take a daily vitamin D supplement to ensure adequate levels throughout the year. Vitamin D3 is the preferred form of supplementation. Vitamin D2, a synthetic version, is not as effective at raising and maintaining blood levels of vitamin D. Use the guidelines in Week 50, Upgrade Your Medicine Cabinet, to find a high-quality supplement manufacturer.

FOSTER A POSITIVE RELATIONSHIP TO FOOD

Your relationship to food is but a reflection of your relationship to yourself, as is everything in your life.

—MARIANNE WILLIAMSON

THE ROLE OF food in our lives is multifaceted. We use food to fuel our bodies, celebrate special occasions, connect with friends and family, commemorate our heritage, and explore new cultures. Food is at the center of how we relate to our world; it's connected to our emotions and interwoven into our memories. As such, the nature of our relationship with food can have a dramatic impact on our ability to enjoy life.

Having a positive relationship with food brings many benefits. Studies by Ellyn Satter, family therapist and registered dietician, show that people who are "positive, comfortable, flexible with eating and reliable about getting enough to eat of enjoyable and nourishing food tend to have better diets, lower BMIs, better physical self acceptance, better medical and lab tests, better sleep, and are more active."[1,2]

YOUR INFLUENCE AS A PARENT

Research shows that the eating habits of our children are a reflection of our own patterns. For example, one study found that children of parents who eat fruit and vegetables every day tend to eat more servings of produce than children with parents who rarely eat fruit and vegetables.[3] Parental influence can have a negative effect on eating behaviors, as well. Restricting food intake, offering treats as a reward, or rewarding healthy eating can backfire in the long term, producing undesired results. For example, a well-known study found that preschool children who were rewarded for various good behaviors with a sweet snack, such as animal crackers, raisins, or vanilla wafers, developed a much stronger preference for sweet snacks.[4] Other studies have shown that children who are rewarded for eating specific foods (such as vegetables) develop less of a preference for the foods eaten to obtain the reward.[5,6]

Many American parents are focused primarily on what children eat. Since we can't truly control this aspect of eating, however, parents easily become stressed. In fact, a survey of two thousand Americans found the most stressful times of the day for parents are mealtimes, especially breakfast and dinner. Parents worry about satisfying everyone's taste buds and how to satisfy finicky eaters.[7] Yet although you can serve healthy food and let children choose from what's served, you can't (and shouldn't) control which of the foods they eat or how much they eat. As with other life skills, children need to learn how to feed themselves. When parents focus on creating a supportive mealtime environment, children are free to develop a joyful and healthy relationship with food and healthy eating habits.

You can help your family develop a healthy attitude toward food by modeling how to enjoy food, teaching them how to identify their hunger and satisfaction cues, and showing them how to find foods they enjoy in any setting. Facilitating a healthy attitude toward food as early as possible will establish eating behaviors that persist into adolescence and adulthood.[8]

DID YOU KNOW?

Children emulate parental attitudes toward food, including dieting and food restriction. One study found that five-year-old girls whose mothers were currently or recently dieting were twice as likely to think about dieting as girls with mothers who did not diet.[9] Another study found that ten-year-old girls of mothers who dieted and had negative feelings about eating were more likely to diet and have negative thoughts about their eating behaviors.[10]

THE CHANGE
FOSTER A POSITIVE RELATIONSHIP WITH FOOD.

PATH TO CHANGE   Use the following techniques to create a supportive eating environment to help children become competent eaters.

MAKE MEALTIMES POSITIVE   Children who experience enjoyable mealtimes create positive associations between meals, food, and family. Yet stressful mealtimes cause cortisol (a stress hormone) levels to rise, creating negative associations with food and eating. Keep discipline out of mealtimes as much as possible to preserve the sacredness of making mealtimes a positive experience. See Week 47, Cook In, Eat Together, for tips on creating a positive experience during family meals.

SOMETHING FOR EVERYONE   Include something in your meal that each person enjoys. While your preschooler may not put your spouse's favorite green bean dish on his plate, he may devour the chicken strips. Let each family member fill up on whatever meal components he or she prefers most. Taking this approach in meal planning allows parents to incorporate new foods on the table without stress or fear. Children may or may not try new foods, but having exposure to lots of new foods or the same foods in different forms eventually increases a child's comfort with a wide variety of foods.

SERVE FAMILY STYLE   Rather than preplating food for your children, allow them to serve themselves from bowls and plates containing the prepared dishes. Serving food family style empowers children to pay attention to their own needs and preferences and provide for themselves in a controlled setting. With time, children learn to eat what their body needs in terms of protein, fat, vegetables, and so on.

Relinquish control Despite good intentions, using obvious control strategies to influence what your child eats or how much he eats has been shown to produce undesired results. For instance, one study showed that when mothers increased the use of control strategies at mealtimes, the level of food neophobia (fear of new foods) in their children increased in the present and persisted for up to two years later.[11] Parental pressures at mealtimes, whether negative or positive in nature, interfere with a child's ability to recognize internal cues such as hunger, fullness, and enjoyment.

Sit and eat together Though the chaos of modern family life may make it seemingly impossible to sit and eat with your family, your presence at the table provides much more than just companionship. Children mimic how parents select foods to eat, test new foods, and recognize internal hunger cues by getting additional helpings of a meal or stopping once full. The more often you eat with your family, the more opportunities you have to model a healthy relationship with food and your body. What's more, creating a ritual of shared meals goes a long way in supporting healthy development of children. Research shows teens who participate in family meals are less likely to abuse substances, engage in violent behavior, experience depression, and practice risky eating behaviors, such as binge eating.[12,13,14] Refer to Week 47, Cook In, Eat Together, for more information on eating together as a family.

PRACTICE MINDFUL EATING STRATEGIES   Mindful eating involves deepening our connection with food and understanding its impact on our body and mind. It includes using all of our senses and taking the time to recognize and respect our food preferences and internal cues regarding hunger and fullness.[15] Some tips:

Remove distractions We eat more when meals are eaten in front of the television, while working, or doing things that disable us from focusing on our internal hunger and satisfaction mechanisms. Eat at the table and avoid distractions so everyone is more aware of personal hunger cues.

Use your senses A baby uses his eyes, fingers, mouth, and even nose to explore food, but this practice can be enjoyed by all ages, as well. Ask children what they notice when exploring their food. Take it one step further and ask how they feel about the food, both emotionally and physically.

SEE AN EATING SPECIALIST   Reversing negative relationships with food can be challenging. Parents who have a positive relationship with food are better at feeding their children and at fostering healthy connections with the food they eat. By adopting the strategies laid out in this chapter, you'll create a positive environment for your children to eat competently. If, however, a child's eating behavior seems impossible to shift, contact a childhood eating specialist. Thousands of nutritionists and eating specialists have helped parents and children improve eating competence, regardless of age.

MAKE SCREEN TIME PURPOSEFUL

The great myth of our times is that
technology is communication.

—Libby Larsen

TECHNOLOGY PERMEATES OUR lives, especially the lives of our children. For decades television was the sole technological audiovisual device we used for entertainment and to detach from society, but today we have a plethora of devices to help us do this: computers, smartphones, tablets, and, of course, TV. While television was used mostly for entertainment, our families now require devices for work, education, and socialization. We use these devices to stay informed, capture memories, and even maintain climate control in our homes.

Although screen use can be necessary, it can mean negative consequences for both mental and physical health. Too much screen time—including television, playing video games, and using computers, smartphones, and tablets—decreases a child's attention span, ability to concentrate, and executive function, while increasing risk of obesity, aggressive behavior, depression, and even loneliness.[1,2,3] And the earlier the exposure, the earlier the problems, including lack of attention span, seem to develop.[4]

While there has been limited research on the use of technology by younger children, we can look to studies on adolescents to understand the impact. For computer and mobile device usage, a study conducted by Sarah Thomée at the University of Gothenburgh found that constant use of computers and mobile devices can lead to stress, sleeping disorders, and depression in young adults.[6] Another review, conducted by Dr. Karen Martin of the University of Western Australia, found that adolescents experience low mood, loneliness, and depression with online social networking and basic internet use.[7] Screen use not only displaces sleep, especially in older children, but also replaces physical activity and movement, both of which are important to maintaining healthy sleep patterns.

Although we feel that technology keeps us "connected," it actually diminishes the quality of our social interactions. For very young children, exposure to screens interferes with brain development, specifically the area of the brain responsible for understanding social cues and responding to nonverbal signs like facial expressions required for developing empathy and compassion. One interesting study evaluated the impact of screen use on attachment to peers and parents by looking at two large groups of adolescents almost sixteen years apart. The study found screen use, with both televisions and computers, was associated with low attachment to parents and peers.[9] Every moment on a screen is one moment less interacting live with family and friends, increasing the risk of depression. A study conducted at the University of Maryland found that unhappy people watch more television, whereas people who describe themselves as "very happy" spend more time reading and socializing.

As your family spends less time in front of a screen, their dependency will wane. Look at this change as an opportunity to help children try new activities, use their imagination, develop a new hobby, or deepen their relationships with friends and family.

TECHNOLOGY AND THE DEMISE OF OUTDOOR PLAYTIME[10]

Over the last twenty years, we have seen a significant decline in the amount of time we spend outdoors. In a survey from Hofstra University, 70 percent of mothers reported playing outside every day when they were young, compared to only 31 percent of their children.

This decline in outdoor playtime can be directly attributed to advances in technology and media. In a study of 8,950 preschoolers, children were exposed to screens for 3.2 to 5.6 hours each day depending upon the type of childcare provided (center-based, parental care, or home-based care).[11] As children grow, the average time spent on screens each day also increases much more than it did in the past.

THE CHANGE
GO ON A SCREEN DETOX.

PATH TO CHANGE It may seem like a daunting task, but all the benefits of reducing screen time make it well worth the effort. Consider the following strategies:

START A DIALOGUE Start communicating with your children about the value of social interactions and time spent on activities that do not require a screen. Help older children identify what they are missing during typical screen time. And, of course, talk about how you will benefit from less screen time, too, so they realize all family members can use a little improvement. As a family, talk about experiences you'd enjoy if screens weren't available.

REDUCE EXPOSURE Many parents are shocked to realize how much screen time their families actually experience each day. The average American youth spends 900 hours in school per year—and 1,200 hours watching television. When you consider time spent on tablets, computers, and mobile devices, this number dramatically rises. Reducing screen time will allow you and your children to spend more time with others, embrace new hobbies or master existing ones, and free up more time for fun and important life experiences. Cancel your cable subscription or downgrade your family's text and data plans. Doing this should raise awareness of time spent texting and web surfing.

Raise awareness Your family likely doesn't realize how much screen time each member experiences each day. For each member of the family, copy the Media Inventory Worksheet in Part III: Tools and Resources to log the hours spent on various devices for school, work, and personal use. When you've completed a week's worth, tally up the hours spent on each device, as well as the total hours spent on all screens per day.

SCREEN TIME GUIDELINES[12,13]

AGE	DAILY SCREEN TIME MAXIMUM
0 to 18 months	*Avoid all screen use*
18 to 24 months	<1 hour of high-quality, educational apps or programs used with an adult
2 to 5 years	<1 hour of high-quality, educational content
6+ years	<2 hours entertainment content

Implement Each day, tally the number of hours of screen time spent and continually work toward meeting goals. When possible, have children do this for themselves. If any family member goes over the maximum on a given day, explore together how to spend less time the next day.

EXPLORE NEW ACTIVITIES Encourage everyone to develop a new hobby or schedule more time with friends. Children are quite resourceful and will find ways to entertain themselves when technology and screens are not an option. Give younger children access to toys and crafts that require imagination, such as magnetic blocks, Tinkertoys, and Play-Doh. Older children may enjoy music, art, books, or sports.

SKIP DIGITAL; GO LIVE INSTEAD Choose to do things in person and without technology. Instead of watching television or a movie, opt for a live performance, such as a play or concert. Look for child-friendly performances at community theatres, schools, and children's theatres. Even adult-oriented venues hold multiple child-friendly performances throughout the year. Choose board games or physical games, such as laser tag or paint ball. And, of course, instead of texting, encourage children to call friends or visit in person.

INTERACTIVE EDUCATION Older children may require time on the computer for school-based projects. Instead of searching the Internet for information, bring children to a library, museum, or business to find information that is relevant to their school assignments.

TECHNOLOGY-FREE DESIGNATIONS

At home Designate certain areas of your home as screen-free zones. This is especially important in the bedroom, as avoiding devices two hours before bedtime is critical for production of melatonin. As we discuss in Week 2, Sleep Soundly, using technology near bedtime keeps the mind wired and unable to settle down for sleep.

Mealtimes Eating in front of a screen, whether it's a television or computer, disrupts the communication between the brain and stomach, making it more difficult to recognize fullness. Research confirms eating in front of a screen regularly increases intake.[14] Help children connect with their food by skipping screens during meals.

Other times Schedule technology-free family time each week to encourage interaction and improve relationships. Hold game nights or visit local attractions together, such as the zoo, museums, or sporting events, or do outdoor activities. During these times, use technology purely for capturing photos in the moment so you can share them later.

SAY NO IN COMPANY   When your family is in the company of others, make a point of turning off all connected devices. Children of all ages develop social skills through live interactions; screens hamper this. If this rule frustrates older children, help them find ways to make socialization in your home more fun. For example, let them blast music and have a dance party, create at-home paint nights, get an air hockey table, or install a basketball hoop.

SAY THANKS

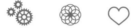

Gratitude is the sign of noble souls.
—AESOP

THANKSGIVING IS THE most common time of year for families to focus on gratitude. Schools and day cares incorporate gratitude-themed projects into curricula. We often see individuals of all ages participating in challenges on social media, highlighting things for which they are thankful. This focus on gratitude is rewarding and brings deeper joy, enthusiasm, and optimism to all who take part. Looking beyond the Thanksgiving holiday, however, and adopting a gratitude-based mindset throughout the year can provide many long-term positive benefits to the well-being of children and adults.

The Youth Gratitude Project (YGP), part of UC Berkeley's Greater Good Science Center, evaluates the scientific components of gratitude and its impact on a child's well-being, as well as how to effectively foster gratitude early in a child's life. In one study, researchers at YGP found adolescents who were more grateful had higher GPAs and life satisfaction and were more socially integrated and less depressed and envious than their less grateful peers.[1] And another YGP study of middle schoolers found that children who learn to be grateful tend to express thanks more often and exhibit a more positive mindset.[2]

Gratitude is more than being thankful; it entails a focus on the joyful aspects of life and the habit of applying positivity to overcome negative experiences. We know that the teenage years can be an emotionally charged period. Unfortunately, recent trends indicate teen depression and anxiety has increased.[3] Teaching teens how to recognize and reframe negative experiences into more positive opportunities is a powerful gratitude-based strategy for developing resiliency and greater life satisfaction. Further, studies show grateful people sleep better, have a stronger immune system, and are less depressed—benefits that everyone, especially teenagers, can appreciate![4,5]

People who feel grateful tend to spread their positivity to people around them, even to strangers.[6] Becoming a family committed to practicing gratitude will have a positive impact on your family and the community around you.

DID YOU KNOW?

A longitudinal study showed teens and tweens who are most grateful are more motivated to find a purpose in life, and connect and contribute to people and society in support of their purpose. This study, conducted by Giacomo Bono and Robert Emmons, professors and leaders of YGP, remind us that instilling gratefulness in children can help them lead a more meaningful life.[7]

THE CHANGE
PRACTICE GRATITUDE.

PATH TO CHANGE Incorporating gratitude-focused behaviors into family life makes the intangible practice of gratitude more concrete to children. Try the following activities with your family:

KEEP GRATITUDE JOURNALS Writing in journals weekly or daily can foster a grateful mindset when we spend time elaborating on the details of what we are thankful for rather than just creating a simple list. You can create a family journal to incorporate everyone's thoughts or keep individual journals. Young children can draw pictures or enlist older siblings and parents to capture their personal perspectives in the journal. Make gratitude journaling a regular family activity by incorporating it into other routines, such as bedtime or before dinner.

MAKE GRATITUDE VISIBLE Retailers stock décor promoting gratitude over the Thanksgiving holiday. Incorporate those signs into your décor throughout the year. Posting reminders to be thankful throughout your home can help older children and adults pause and reflect. For younger children, use chalkboards to create and display new items of thanks— update it each month!

RANDOM ACTS OF GRATITUDE Spread gratitude to friends and family, and even strangers, by creating offers of thanks throughout the year. Make cookies for local police and fire departments. Send thank-you cards to friends for their friendship. Work as a family to cowrite letters of gratitude to a family member or create pictures of thanks. Performing these random acts of thanks can be a fun, exciting way for children to share gratitude authentically.

SAVOR THE GOOD IN LIFE Spend a few moments each day appreciating the goodness in the day. This can be routine, especially for younger children, or a spontaneous discussion. Model for children how to appreciate simple pleasures such as the first sight of spring flowers or birds chirping. Spend more time discussing the positive rather than the negative aspects of your day with your family. You can prompt children to do the same, using purposeful questions such as "What did someone share with you today?" or "What made you laugh today?"

CELEBRATE LOUD AND PROUD   Shout from the mountaintops when good things, big and small, happen to you or your family members. By celebrating the good in life, we focus our energy on the positive, thereby naturally teaching children how to embrace goodness and articulate appreciation. Celebrations need not be extravagant, but could include a balloon, handpicked flowers, handmade cards, or a simple family toast to mark the occasion.

VERBALIZE GRATITUDE TO LOVED ONES   Make it a priority to tell your loved ones how much you appreciate them. Expressing thanks for the little things they do and the big projects they take on makes them feel supported, acknowledged, and loved. Teach your children that although we don't mean to, it's common to take our loved ones for granted. Make it a habit to verbalize gratitude by establishing routines for sharing thanks with each other, such as over breakfast or dinner.

TEACH REFRAMING   Using gratitude to reframe negative experiences helps children build resiliency. When something bad happens to children, parents can start by acknowledging the child's hurt feelings, an act that establishes security and trust and reinforces empathy. On the other hand, stewing in negativity brings children down. Teach children how to find the positive or the opportunity in a negative situation. For young children, it can be as simple (and silly) as pointing out that a dropped ice cream cone provides unexpected food for ants!

REFLECT ON GRACIOUS ACTS   You can help children truly understand what gratitude means by using the Deepening Gratitude worksheet found in Part III: Tools and Resources. Use it when someone shows kindness to your child or gives him a gift. The exercise prompts reflection and discussion by having you ask a few key questions to help your child discover gratitude more deeply.[8] In one study, the benefits appraisal was used as a tool to teach gratitude to elementary school students. After using it, students reported more positive emotions and exhibited more grateful behaviors immediately, and up to five months after the exercise.[9]

BUST A MOVE

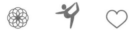

We do not stop exercising because we grow old—
we grow old because we stop exercising.

—Dr. Kenneth Cooper

IT'S NO SECRET: exercise and physical activity are crucial for optimal health of both adults and children. People who exercise regularly have a lower incidence of heart disease, stroke, depression, type 2 diabetes, and some cancers.[1] Exercise reduces stress and decreases inflammation. It lowers blood sugar because muscles use energy from food without producing insulin. It also supports a strong immune system, healthy brain function, and the development and maintenance of strong bones and muscles. You are never too young or too old to benefit from increased physical activity and exercise.

Fortunately, young children are naturally very active when given the opportunity. But, as children reach ages nine to twelve, studies indicate physical activity tends to decrease, even in active children.[2] Exercise can actually ease the physical and psychological changes that children of this age commonly experience from hormone surges associated with puberty. For example, studies show exercise supports a healthy weight, improves self-esteem, helps manage anxiety and stress, promotes healthy sleep, and lowers the incidence of depression in children and adolescents.[3,4]

YOUR INFLUENCE AS A PARENT

Now more than ever, exercise is an imperative for children, as experts find this generation of children is the most sedentary in history! Studies show, however, that parents can have a huge impact on this statistic. One study found children with parents who encouraged activity and interacted with them actively were six times more likely to be highly active than inactive.[5] And moms who model healthy physical activity have an especially influential role in boosting the activity of kids.[6]

Being active together helps children develop habits and behaviors that extend into adulthood. It can also motivate parents who have a tough time prioritizing physical activity for their own personal health, because, whether we like it or not, our children can be diligent about ensuring we stick to our commitments. Your family can benefit from any increase in movement, be it performing structured exercise together, such as cycling, fitness classes, and running, or just walking and swimming more regularly.

DID YOU KNOW?

Children who are physically fit are more likely to have better grades and stronger academic performance. Many factors are at play, but one study by researchers at the University of Illinois showed that the brain neurons of active children fired more quickly and strongly than those of inactive children.[7]

THE CHANGE
GET MOVING TOGETHER.

PATH TO CHANGE   Physical activity provides numerous benefits to the whole family. Use the following techniques to create healthy activity behaviors that last a lifetime:

MAKE FAMILY TIME ACTIVE   Replace time watching movies and television with fun physical movement. Use pre- or post-dinner walks to reflect on each other's day and talk about life. Instill pride in children by doing physical household projects together, such as planting flowers, raking leaves, shoveling, or washing the car. Schedule adventures to explore your region on bikes, kayaks, or canoes. Let children help select and plan some projects and adventures to increase their interest and mood during active family time!

PRIORITIZE MOVEMENT   Evenings and weekends can get filled up quickly with homework, afterschool activities, chores, and birthday parties. When physical activity isn't prioritized and planned, it often goes by the wayside during busy times. Schedule specific days and times for your family's physical activity. When other commitments threaten these protected times, be sure to reschedule family movement instead of canceling it altogether.

PROVIDE ACTIVE TOYS   Boost the fun in your activity with developmentally appropriate active toys. Use balls to play sports together, like soccer, basketball, kickball, and dodgeball. Build leg and core strength with jump ropes, trampolines, and pogo sticks. Add an element of fun to summer events by including beach paddles, badminton, and other back-and-forth games.

PRACTICE SPORTS   Whether you grew up playing a sport or not, playing sports with your children can have a long-term effect. Research shows children at age ten who are active in sports, more so than neighborhood outdoor play, become more active adults.[8] Give your younger children opportunities to try many different sports so they are more likely to find something they enjoy. Enlist tips from coaches on how to teach new skills at home and then work together on technique. You'll have fun without any pressure, and your child will have fun because you've taken an interest in a sport he loves.

EXPLORE NEW ACTIVITIES Seek out new activities to try together as a family. Indoor rock climbing is a big trend and can safely be practiced by children as young as age three. Try acroyoga, a form of the ancient practice that will have your family flipping like acrobats. There are plenty of activities to try. You may love some and vow never to repeat others. Enjoy the exploration and the opportunity to move your bodies in healthy ways as a family.

USE TECHNOLOGY It may seem counterintuitive, but using technology to boost physical activity can be quite effective. For example, one study showed people who received updates via social media on the physical activity of their peer networks increased their own physical activity moderately for an additional 1.6 days, on average.[9] Another study found that sending text messages to teens promoting the enjoyment associated with physical activity boosted their activity by an additional two hours per week![10]

DO IT FOR CHARITY Throughout the year, you're sure to find plenty of walks, bike rides, or runs dedicated to raising money for charity. Find a family-friendly event connected to a cause your family finds important, and commit to participation as a team. You'll have fun practicing for the event while also boosting your movement. For adults and children alike, setting physical activity goals that culminate in celebrations adds an element of fun that may not otherwise exist.

BEYOND SPORTS

USE THE FOLLOWING tips to help your children increase their movement and exercise naturally through regular play or scheduled activities.

AGE	STRATEGIES
Preschool (3 to 6 years)	**MAKE IT A GAME!** Children learn through play, so promote movement as part of your play together. Games like tag, hide and seek, and cops and robbers are sure to get them engaged. **CONNECT WITH THEIR INTERESTS!** Create your play around a theme that makes your child's heart sing, whether it is nature, superheroes, or princesses!
Tweens (7 to 12 years)	**THINK BEYOND SPORTS!** Not everyone is interested in organized, team-based sports. This age is the perfect time to get your child to try other activities, such as yoga, dance, or parkour. It's important your child has fun, so if she loses interest, try another activity.
Teens (13 to 17 years)	**MAKE IT FUN AND AGE APPROPRIATE!** At this age, teens can participate in structured exercise, including fitness classes and weight lifting. Bring teens with you to spin class, Zumba, or CrossFit, or sign up for personal training sessions together!

EAT THE RAINBOW

An apple a day keeps the doctor away.
—BENJAMIN FRANKLIN

NO DOUBT, FRUITS and vegetables are good for you and your family. Fresh produce is packed with vitamins, minerals, fiber, and phytonutrients—powerful compounds that not only give plants their color (and in some cases protect them from predation), but also protect humans against diseases such as cancer, diabetes, and heart disease. The health benefits of consuming fruits and vegetables are well documented and universally accepted. Yet produce intake of both adults and children in America is far below where it should be.

A study by the Centers for Disease Control (CDC) found that 60 percent of children and 18 percent of adults are not eating enough fruit each day, and the diets of 93 percent of children and 86 percent of adults are missing adequate vegetables.[1] Most adults freely admit their produce consumption is far from adequate, but even those following a healthy diet may still fall shy of ideal intake.

According to the latest research, the USDA recommendation of four to six servings of produce daily is far too conservative to achieve protective health benefits. In a massive study of over sixty-five thousand people, researchers found consuming more than seven servings of fruits and vegetables daily reduces a person's risk of death from all causes by at least 23 percent. For people who live a sedentary life or have smoked in their lifetime, the benefit doubles, with the risk of death reduced by 48 percent.[2] Another study found that people who ate eight or more servings of produce daily reduced their risk of heart attack or stroke by 30 percent.[3] Authorities on nutrition, including the Institute for Functional Medicine and the Cleveland Clinic, recommend that people consume seven to ten servings of fruits and vegetables per day, with an emphasis on nonstarchy vegetables.

POWERFUL PRODUCE

Overall, a diet filled with fruits and vegetables of all different colors of the rainbow is most protective against disease and death. Here are a few star players:

Cruciferous vegetables (such as broccoli): contain high levels of glucosinolates, sulfur-containing compounds critical for detoxification of harmful substances, which protect against cancers of the bladder, breast, colon, gastrointestinal organs, lungs, ovaries, pancreas, prostate, and kidneys.

Berries: rich in antioxidants such as vitamin C, polyphenols, and flavonoids that reduce oxidative stress and inflammation, and anthocyanins, compounds that lower blood pressure and improve the elasticity of blood vessels.

Nitric oxide–rich vegetables (such as beets): powered by nitric oxide, a potent vasodilator (opens your blood vessels) shown to lower blood pressure and improve vascular function.[4,5,6,7]

YOUR INFLUENCE AS A PARENT

Parental modeling is by far one of the most effective strategies at helping shape our children's eating patterns. Though young children may find some vegetables, such as Brussels sprouts, less desirable than cucumbers or sweet potatoes, research shows that the more exposure children have to foods, the more food rejection will dissipate. Overall, produce consumption is highest in households where parents eat lots of fruits and vegetables, make produce easily accessible, and prepare it in delicious ways.

DID YOU KNOW?

To grow enough fruits and vegetables for Americans to eat the USDA's daily intake recommendation, "the supply of fruit would need to double" and "the supply of vegetables would need to increase by 70 percent with nearly all of the increase coming from dark green vegetables and legumes."[8] Current government policy and subsidies encourage production of corn, soy, and wheat instead of fruits and vegetables.

THE CHANGE
EAT SEVEN OR MORE SERVINGS OF PRODUCE EVERY DAY.

PATH TO CHANGE   American vegetable consumption tend to focus on tomatoes and potatoes—a diet that's missing thousands of disease-fighting phytonutrients. Use the following tips to boost your family's health with a wider variety of produce:

FILL HALF THE PLATE For every meal and snack, aim to include half a plate of colorful produce, a simple yet effective strategy for eating seven servings daily. Keep in mind, serving food family style is a tried-and-true approach for raising healthy, competent eaters (see Week 7, Foster a Positive Relationship to Food). It's easy to follow this approach when packing school lunches and snacks for your children. At other meals, adults can simply model this approach when filling their own plate with food.

MAKE IT TASTY Taste is by far the most important reason people choose one food over another, especially children. You don't have to be a professional chef to make delicious fruit- and vegetable-based meals. Fruit in peak season is juicy, sweet, and easy to love with simple preparation. Vegetables can be prepared in ways that enhance their flavor and make them addictive! Here are a few options for getting started:

Ice pops Transform smoothies into a kid-friendly favorite by simply freezing them into molds. Traditional ice pop molds are inexpensive and take three to four hours to freeze. Zoku is a new ice pop product that can create pops in just seven to nine minutes! In the summer, serve them at breakfast, as a snack, or for dessert.

Juice it Fruit juice is very high in sugar, even when made at home. Instead, make juice with lots of vegetables and add a small amount of fruit. Choose cold-pressed juicers for getting the most juice from your produce. Some nutrients break down when exposed to light and air, so it is ideal to drink freshly made green juice. If juicing at home isn't an option, fresh juice companies are becoming more and more popular in cities and surrounding areas. Or you can purchase cold-pressed bottled juice produced by reputable companies such as Suja (www.sujajuice.com) or Here (www.here.co).

Smoothies When prepared without added sugar, smoothies are a very nutritious option that packs in a lot of produce. The best smoothies are made with a high-speed blender such as a Ninja or Vitamix, but any blender will do. Before experimenting on your own, start with a well-tested ratio of 1 cup leafy greens, 1 cup liquid, and 1½ cups of fruit. Blend the greens and liquid first to reduce any leaf particles. Then add a mix of frozen fruit and fresh or thawed fruit to make it sweet. Make it a meal by adding protein and healthy fat such as hemp seeds and avocado, or nut butter. Mix and match ingredients from the following chart to create new colors of the rainbow:

ADD-INS	OPTIONS
Liquid bases	Unsweetened plant-based milk such as almond, coconut, cashew, or hemp Liquefied cucumber Unsweetened coconut water Water
Fruits	Apple, banana, berries, cherries, grapes, mango, peach, pear, pineapple
Greens	Arugula, cabbage, chard, dandelion, kale, romaine, spinach
Fats and proteins	Hemp seeds, nut butters, coconut oil, chia seeds, flax seeds, avocado
Herbs (optional)	Basil, mint, parsley
Spices and flavors (optional)	Cinnamon, ginger, turmeric, cacao powder, maca powder

Roasted To roast vegetables, first cut them into similar-size pieces. Smaller sizes cook more quickly than larger sizes (but if too small, they can burn). Then give them a light drizzle of extra-virgin olive oil and toss in a bowl to ensure they are all coated evenly. Be careful not to use too much oil or the veggies will become greasy. Spread them out on a sheet pan so the pieces have plenty of space to cook evenly and roast properly. Roast at 425°F (220°C) for 15 to 45 minutes, depending on the vegetable (check on them every 15 minutes). This higher temperature often browns them on the outside, making them especially delicious.

Steamed and dressed To make steamed vegetables more palatable and less bland, toss veggies in a simple dressing. A few delicious combinations include: maple syrup and extra-virgin olive oil; honey and mustard; lemon and extra-virgin olive oil.

Pickled Many children love pickles. The good news is, any vegetable can be pickled! Vinegar-based pickled vegetables are the most common because they are shelf stable. Fermented pickled vegetables, however, are the most nutritious versions because the process promotes the proliferation of beneficial bacteria called probiotics. Look for them in the refrigerated section of your grocery store and check the label to ensure they contain live bacteria. Fermented vegetables last two to three months after opening when kept in the fridge.

Stir-fry/sauté Prepare vegetables in a sauté pan with a bit of extra-virgin olive oil and salt for a simple and quick alternative to roasting.

COLORFUL APPETIZERS   Serve sliced raw veggies as appetizers before dinner. Parents can prepare dinner without children whining about hunger, and kids can get another healthy serving of veggies. Serve a couple of different color veggies to make the dish more eye-pleasing, and cut veggies in different ways so children get curious about what's on the plate.

FRUIT FOR DESSERT   When in season, fruit is naturally sweet and makes for a delicious dessert. Chop up fruit, and if your little one has a sweeter palate, drizzle with honey. Or put fresh fruit on a skewer to make it extra fun. Roast fruit with cinnamon and honey for an extra flavorful twist.

JUST BREATHE

Every breath we take, every step we make,
can be filled with peace, joy, and serenity.

—THICH NHAT HANH

WITH ROOTS DATING back five thousand years, the ancient practice of meditation is no longer reserved for Buddhist monks and hippies. It is a powerful tool used by people from all walks of life: from Olympians and business moguls to elementary school students and truck drivers. In the United States, more than 18,000,000 adults and 900,000 children have tried meditation—a number that continues to grow rapidly.[1,2] People who practice meditation experience a sense of calm, peace, psychological balance, and mental focus, even after the meditation session is over.

Research on the health benefits of meditation is extensive and well recognized by both conventional medicine and alternative health practitioners. Meditation calms the mind and helps us simply observe and release distracting thoughts, resulting in enhanced focus and concentration. Meditation is also useful in managing stress and achieving a deeper feeling of well-being and positivity. It has been used to reduce blood pressure; prevent and treat anxiety, depression, and insomnia; and manage chronic pain. Studies show that for people with mild to moderate anxiety or depression, meditation is as effective as an antidepressant.[3] Meditation also helps reduce inflammation and strengthens the immune system response against pathogens—bacteria or viruses that can cause disease.[4]

Children who practice meditation experience improved focus and attention, reduced anxiety, reduced impulsiveness, lower levels of stress, and better emotional control. In one study, a school-based program of mindful awareness practice (MAP) heavily focused on meditation was implemented in four separate classrooms of second and third graders in Los Angeles, California. Children participated in program activities for just thirty minutes, twice per week for eight weeks. At the end of the program, both teachers and parents reported improvements in the children's executive functioning, including behavior regulation, metacognition, and overall global executive control. What's more, the children with the greatest improvements had been identified as least regulated before the training.[5] For similar reasons, meditation is also used as a complementary therapy to help those with ADHD and attention problems. Fortunately, children whose parents use complementary health tools, such as meditation, are more likely to use them as well.[6]

DID YOU KNOW?

Meditation changes your brain. Research shows meditating as a regular habit increases gray matter in the hippocampus and other brain structures associated with learning and memory, while decreasing the density of gray matter in the amygdala, which is associated with stress.[7,8]

THE CHANGE
INCORPORATE MEDITATION INTO YOUR DAILY ROUTINE.

PATH TO CHANGE A meditation practice of only ten minutes a day can help your family feel grounded and emotionally balanced. Incorporating meditation into your family's typical routine will make it easier for every-one to stay committed—even young children will look forward to medita-tion time. Use the following tips to get started:

STRUCTURE YOUR PRACTICE   Find a specific day and time to meditate. Meditation can be done at any time of the day, but you may find it espe-cially beneficial to practice early in the morning before the day begins or at night to end your day. Once your family decides when to practice, you'll want to choose a style, location, and duration to get started.

Select a style There are many types of meditation, and no single style is better than another. Some people may find moving during meditation easier; others find focusing on the breath to be more relaxing. Finding the right style for each family member will lead to higher success with adopting a meditation habit.

FOUR MEDITATION STYLES

STYLE	DESCRIPTION
Concentrative	Requires focus on something such as your breath or an image. Start by getting comfortable and then begin focusing on your breathing. Notice how your breathing is automatic and how your belly expands and contracts with each breath. When thoughts come into your head, take notice and release them as you return to your breath.
Guided	Requires listening to a live person or a recorded voice to guide you in meditation. Instructors will remind you to bring your attention back to the meditation and will keep track of the time. Beginners often appreciate the ease of guided meditation.
Mantra-based	Similar to concentrative meditation, you will focus on a specific mantra to keep your attention. You can choose the mantra, such as "I am strong," to repeat over and over silently to yourself.
Movement-based	Meditating in action (such as during walking, yoga, or tai chi) is effective as long as you keep your focus on your body, rather than on the world around you. For example, in a walking meditation, start by focusing on how your feet hit the ground, how they feel in your shoes, what feels different when they walk over bumps or crunchy leaves, how your ankles connect to your feet, and whether they feel tight or relaxed.

Choose a spot Find a place that is conducive to quiet and has limited distractions, especially if children are participating. This may be in a quiet room in your home or a nearby peaceful park. If practicing a seated meditation, make sure everyone has a comfortable place to sit or lie down, such as on a bench, chair, pillow, or blanket. For moving meditation, find plenty of space to move without distraction.

Get comfortable Wear comfortable clothing that isn't too restrictive, especially when sitting in the same spot for five to twenty minutes. Also, add or remove layers to find a comfortable temperature. Seated meditation is traditionally performed sitting upright in a cross-legged position, but children might find it easier to lie down or lean against a wall for support.

Be patient Start with just five minutes of dedicated time daily. Check in with your family after each session and discuss increasing your time commitment. Although research shows that twenty minutes of meditation, practiced two times per day, produces the most health benefits, positive results can be seen with just ten minutes daily.

USE TECHNOLOGY   From podcasts to apps, there are many ways technology can enhance your meditation practice. Guided meditation or meditative music is available on iTunes and Amazon. Many meditation teachers offer podcast series of guided meditations that you can listen to on your phone, tablet, or computer. Children's meditation apps are worthwhile because of all of the content.

TAKE A MEDITATION WORKSHOP   Yoga studios, mind/body centers, public libraries, and wellness centers have started offering meditation workshops. Workshops vary in length and may focus on different meditation styles. Instructors provide guided meditations and gear workshops to each participant's level of experience with meditation. You'll often leave a workshop feeling refreshed and very comfortable with adopting a meditation practice at home. Many workshops will allow older children and teenagers to participate, as well; check with the instructor.

LET YOUR IMAGINATION RUN WILD

Every child is an artist; the problem is how
to remain an artist once we grow up.

—PABLO PICASSO

ARTISTIC AND CREATIVE expression benefits the mind and nurtures
the soul. Family members don't need to consider themselves artists to
experience the positive results of cultivating creativity. For example,
researchers reviewed studies that used art, writing, music, and theatre
for the purposes of healing (not mastery) and found that these creative
activities reduced participants' stress, anxiety, depression, and negative
emotions. The review also showed improvements in self-image, positive
emotions, and even physical function when practicing movement-based
activities.[1] Other studies show engaging in creative activities keeps the
mind resilient and provides a sense of control that has a protective effect
against dementia and cognitive decline.[2]

For children, creativity provides a healthy opportunity for inventiveness,
risk taking, self-expression, and problem solving. Building a structure,
writing a play, or designing jewelry requires a child to make constant
decisions without knowing the outcome or whether each step will produce the intended result. This process teaches flexibility and openness

to what may unfold during the creative process and helps children build self-confidence and resilience when things do not go as planned.

Further, skills honed during creative activities support the development of children at all ages. Toddlers and preschoolers use art and building activities to develop language and strengthen motor skills. Children (and adults) express emotions they're not able or ready to communicate in words through creative expression. In one study, children with chronic asthma participated weekly in sixty minutes of art activities designed to encourage expression, problem solving, and discussion in relation to living with asthma. After seven weeks, study participants showed improvements in communications, problem solving, and quality of life, and a decrease in worry and anxiety.[3] For older children, involvement in the arts is associated with educational benefits such as improved academic outcomes, increased standardized test scores, and lower dropout rates.[4] Performing arts involving others, such as dance, music, and theatre, also promote community and the creation of a positive social network that provides children and adolescents a sense of belonging, safety, and security.

Parents can model and prioritize creative exploration for the family. Whether it be cooking, painting, or constructing with LEGOs, the creative process takes your mind off the more strenuous demands of life. These types of quiet activities also open up space in busy lives to process emotions and connect with feelings that may be difficult to face. Finally, creative activities can evolve into lifelong hobbies that make life richer and more meaningful and can even hone problem-solving and innovation skills for current or future careers.

DID YOU KNOW?

According to the 2016 Future of Jobs Report by the World Economic Forum, employers and industry experts named "creativity" as one of the top three skills needed for employees to be successful and qualified for jobs available in the year 2020.[5]

THE CHANGE
MAKE TIME FOR CREATIVE EXPRESSION.

PATH TO CHANGE   Creativity can be expressed through more common practices such as painting, photography, writing, cooking, knitting, and singing, and less common pursuits such as jewelry making, glass blowing, and robotics. Find creative outlets each family member can enjoy and prioritize time for them with the following tips:

DEDICATE A SPACE   Designate an inspirational place, free of distractions, inside or outside your home that allows for complete immersion in the creative process. Ensure there is space for storing supplies, equipment, and tools specific to the activities you want to enjoy, such as art materials, a music stand, an easel, or a tripod. If space is limited, store all of your creative equipment in a metal cart with wheels so it is easily accessible and movable by all family members.

ART AND MESS   Many parents are reluctant to encourage art activities at home because they dread the potential mess. It's no fun to be told you can paint but you must not get paint anywhere except on the paper. Try to embrace the mess and consider it as part of the creative process. You can easily protect floors and furniture with drop cloths, plastic tablecloths, flattened cardboard boxes, and the like.

GET ORGANIZED   Creative exploration may require supplies or equipment, depending on the activity. For example, if your family enjoys traditional art activities, stock up on basic supplies, such as paint, brushes, sponges, colored pencils, and quality paper. Or, if jewelry making, knitting, or robotics is preferred, buy a few kits and appropriate tools so creation can happen spontaneously. You can also get recommendations from staff at Michaels, a national art supply store, or a local art store on types of creative art projects and relevant supplies.

MAKE TIME FOR CREATIVITY   Choose a day and time each week dedicated for creative exploration. For example, mother and children's art teacher Awbree Caton, owner of Bunkhouse Creative, suggests setting out different creative materials a few mornings each week for children to explore before school. Alternatively, devote a couple of hours on a Sunday morning to write, knit, play musical instruments, build, or paint. Creatively inclined parents who spend time on their favorite activities while in the company of family, rather than alone, are more likely to inspire children to participate or be creative, as well.

HAVE A CREATIVE MINDSET   Creativity can happen anytime, anywhere, and doesn't require you to produce a finished product. Musicians jam to explore new chords and sounds. Dancers dance freestyle to explore new steps and practice old moves. Provide your family opportunities to create freely without any restrictions. Skip the coloring books and opt instead for plain white or construction paper. When cooking, focus on the ingredients and flavors desired instead of a recipe. Finally, avoid unintentionally stifling creativity and self-expression. For example, asking, "What did you make or draw?" can send children a message that they should create something recognizable. Instead, comment on the colors, shapes, and function of objects to engage in discussion without providing limitations or labels.

PROMOTE CREATIVE PLAY   For families who may not enjoy visual art or the performing arts, find toys and gadgets that engage the young mind creatively. Refer to the following Creative Toys/Gadgets by Age chart for some ideas.

CREATIVE TOYS/GADGETS BY AGE

AGE	TOYS/GADGETS
1 to 3 years	Wood blocks, DUPLOs, chunky puzzles, plastic measuring cups, stainless steel bowls and wooden spoons, sandboxes
4 to 6 years	Lincoln Logs, LEGOs, Tinkertoys, Squigz, bristle blocks, floor puzzles, gears, Etch A Sketch, kids' musical instruments, Magna-Tiles, sandboxes
7 to 10 years	LEGOs, jewelry-making kits, quilt-making, sewing machine, wood marble runs, puzzles, gears, Squigz, Cranium (the game)
11 to 13 years	Circuit-making kits, model transportation vehicles, mechanical building kits (including pulleys, cranks), 500+ piece puzzles, Cranium
14+ years	Nanoblocks, K'nex kits

LET THEM BE BORED   Children nowadays participate in loads of organized activities and sports, leaving them little unstructured time. Boredom provides space to create. Try not to feel pressure to fill a child's time, but instead let kids explore their own creative interests and passions. Younger children may need more guidance and direction to get started.

CREATIVE ACTIVITIES OUTSIDE THE HOME   Look at local venues and events to participate in preorganized creative activities. Some suggestions include:

- Pottery painting shops
- Jewelry-making classes (try Michaels)
- Knitting or needlepoint classes (try Joann Fabrics)
- Woodworking projects (try Home Depot)
- Family theatre performances

CONSIDER CREATIVE THERAPY   Psychotherapists use music, art, and performance to support children and adults in expressing emotions and feelings associated with trauma, illness, or stress. If someone in your family is having emotional or psychological challenges, consider finding a creative therapist to provide support.

SET GOALS

*The trouble with not having a goal is that
you can spend your life running up and
down the field and never score.*

—BILL COPELAND

SETTING GOALS GIVES you clarity about what you want out of life and provides direction for how you spend your time. But, more important, people who set goals have a higher likelihood of being successful. In their research, Dr. Edwin Locke and Dr. Gary Lantham, pioneers of our modern understanding of goal setting, found that setting goals creates motivation, and when people set personal goals, their performance and success improve.[1]

Various surveys find that less than half the American population sets financial goals or even annual health goals.[2,3] And only 40 percent of Americans create New Year's resolutions or goals for the upcoming year.[4] Yet there's great evidence that goal setting provides many benefits. Setting and achieving goals, no matter how small, elicits positive emotions, such as joy, pride, and a sense of accomplishment. And with achievement you are more motivated to seek even bigger, more challenging goals. What's more, the confidence you develop with goal setting helps quash negative thinking, doubt, and fear, enabling a more positive outlook and a can-do attitude.

At work, setting personalized goals is empowering and results in a deeper sense of ownership of behaviors and work performed. Similarly, students who set their own goals are more self-directed in their learning and experience higher achievement. For example, a randomized study found that struggling undergraduate students who participated in a goal-setting program over a period of four months increased their GPA, had a higher probability of maintaining a full course load, and reported fewer negative feelings.[5] Another study found that undergraduate students who set goals tied to a specific task were more likely to get a grade of B+ or higher in the class than those students who did not set task-specific goals.[6] In primary and secondary school, children learn to set educational goals, but these goals are typically specific to each class and are not personalized. Setting goals at home teaches children personal advocacy, helps them imagine a future they want to create, and reinforces their personal responsibility in creating the life and success they desire.

DID YOU KNOW?

The practice of setting New Year's resolutions can be traced back at least four thousand years. Every year in March (not January), the ancient Babylonians held celebrations and made promises to the gods to repay their debts in return for good fortune in the upcoming year.[7]

THE CHANGE
MAKE GOAL SETTING A FAMILY AFFAIR.

PATH TO CHANGE   Setting goals is a valuable habit to begin at a young age. Use the following strategies to begin:

START SMALL   Big, lofty goals are inspirational, but they take much more time to achieve. By reaching for smaller goals, achievable in the foreseeable future, you can more quickly experience a sense of achievement and the happiness it brings. Small wins can also serve as a motivational tool to push forward on the path toward a much bigger, loftier goal. When setting smaller goals, you can either break a bigger goal down into smaller chunks or set individual smaller goals.

SET BIG GOALS   In his book *Built to Last,* Jim Collins coined the expression "big hairy audacious goals (BHAGs)" to represent goals that are outrageous, energizing, bold, and transformative. BHAGs are inspiring; they force a business or person to consider their capabilities. BHAGs can't be accomplished in five years; they are more like lifelong dreams. Though their completion is far off, BHAGs can serve as a guide for how each family member spends his or her time. For example, if your child sets a goal to compete in a national dance competition, she may discover she'll need to spend a lot more of her time practicing dance, improving her skills, and competing locally.

GET PERSONAL   Effective goals should align with the goal setter's interests, passions, and beliefs. Setting goals authentic to you increases a sense of personal responsibility and ownership over success and failure. The same goes for children's goals—avoid trying to set goals for your children, but instead model and guide them on how to set goals that are authentic to them. Learning to set goals to please oneself versus others helps children become more independent and self-directed.

SAMPLE AGE-APPROPRIATE GOALS FOR CHILDREN:

AGE RANGE	SAMPLE GOAL
3 to 6 years	I will choose a LEGO Juniors set today and use the directions to build it myself. I'll ask Mom and Dad for help only after I have tried myself.
7 to 10 years	I will reduce my screen time outside of school to one hour per day by June. I will put that time toward trying other activities, such as soccer, kung fu, and choir; spend more time with friends; and be active.
11 to 14 years	I will compete in the statewide gymnastics competition this March. I will practice my routines two hours per day, six days a week.
15 to 18 years	I will get my driver's license by the end of the year. I will go to driver's education class in May, and practice driving with Mom and Dad three times per week from May through September.

CONNECT TO A PURPOSE   Setting goals with no clear purpose is an exercise in futility. Attaching a meaningful purpose to your goals is motivating and pushes you through any unforeseeable setbacks. For example, individuals who want to lose weight because their doctor told them it is good for their health may find it difficult to do so. On the other hand, a grandmother who wants to lose weight because she wants to have energy to play with her grandchildren may be more motivated and, as a result, more successful. To find a deeper purpose for your goals, ask your family questions, such as "What will be different if you achieve your goal?" or "How will your life change?" or "What is most exciting about achieving the goal?"

MAKE YOUR GOALS SMARTER   Many experts advise goals should be SMART—specific, measurable, actionable, relevant, and time-bound. Improve your success by setting goals that are also "Emotionally" inspiring and "Readjustable" to increase the likelihood of success. Use the SMARTER Goals Worksheet in Part III: Tools and Resources to guide you in making your goals.

DOCUMENT YOUR GOALS Research shows that individuals who document and share their goals are more likely to be successful than those who don't. Use a chalkboard for capturing family goals or a notebook for goal discussions over dinnertime. Use the SMARTER Goals Worksheet in Part III: Tools and Resources to help your family keep track of goals.

TRACK PROGRESS Keep track of how your family members are doing. That way you can help one another overcome challenges or find motivation on a tough day. Let each family member decide how to track individual progress. For example, young children may enjoy using stickers to celebrate their achievements, while older children may like to track progress on a worksheet attached to the fridge. Reinforce that tracking progress is not about "winning" or "losing" but about celebrating the milestones and effort put forward in reaching goals.

GET INSPIRED Read stories and books about setting goals that appeal to the interests of your family. Some examples: perseverance of athletes, students, musicians, and more.

PRACTICE AND REPEAT Make goal setting a regular practice in your household. Although goals may not always be achieved, setting them regularly helps us become more motivated, focused, and organized in our actions. When failure occurs, see it as an opportunity to learn and grow, and become better at setting goals within reach.

KNOW YOUR FARMER

We have to bring children into a new relationship to food that connects them to culture and agriculture.

—Alice Waters

MUCH OF THE produce found in your neighborhood grocery store has typically traveled thousands of miles, sometimes even across continents, before it reaches your hands. These fruits and vegetables are picked well before ripeness to ensure they'll stay fresh for you to buy. Sadly, this can take a toll on the nutrient retention of your food. For example, one study found broccoli lost 50 percent of its vitamin C after just five days of cold storage post-harvest, and spinach lost 22 percent of lutein after eight days in well-lit storage.[1]

But there is another way! Consuming food grown locally ensures higher nutrient retention in the foods you eat, while also benefiting and stimulating the local economy through local job creation and by keeping money within your community.

Farm-to-school programs, designed to connect children to local food sources, are growing rapidly across the United States. This dynamic programming teaches children about agriculture, offers hands-on projects through gardening, and provides access to nutritious food. Outcomes of these programs include increased consumption of fruits and vegetables, higher willingness to try new foods, and more requests for fruits and vegetables to be served at home.[2,3,4,5] Children who participate in a school garden program, one of the many farm-to-school programming strategies, deepen their knowledge of healthy foods and connection to the earth. Even if your child's school does not yet participate in these programs, the same benefits can be extended to your family through a home garden or a local community garden or by connecting with local farms.

DID YOU KNOW?

Members of CSA (community supported agriculture) programs eat more vegetables and a greater variety, according to a large survey on CSA members in the Central Coast of California conducted by the Center for Agroecology and Sustainable Food Systems at the University of California Santa Cruz.[6]

Gardening can provide benefits of improved nutrition, physical activity, and even social and emotional well-being. Gardening projects give children the opportunity to develop patience and nurturing tendencies, as well as a sense of responsibility. For example, an evaluation of four youth gardening programs for children ages fourteen to nineteen in Colorado found "young gardening participants report feeling calm, happy, relaxed and competent while gardening."[7] Adults and children alike benefit—emotionally, nutritionally, and physically—from growing food together.

THE CHANGE
EAT FOOD GROWN LOCALLY.

PATH TO CHANGE   Eating locally grown food offers health benefits to your family and can also support the local economy. Use the following tips to establish a connection between your family and your food:

JOIN A CSA   Community supported agriculture, or CSA, is a membership-based approach to getting access to local produce, meat, and/or dry goods. Families who join get regular shares of goods grown by one or more local farms. Most local farms now participate in CSAs because they provide more steady and guaranteed income for farmers.

SHOP AT THE FARMERS MARKET   Farmers markets are one of the oldest mechanisms for farmers to connect directly to consumers. As of 2014, over 8,268 farmers markets were operating around the United States.[8] With 180+ percent growth in the past ten years, farmers markets have evolved into fun family events. Markets often include produce, meat, dairy, honey, and dry goods from local farms. And some of the larger markets also allow you to buy wares from local craftspeople, artists, and merchants; see performances by local musicians and community theatres; or participate in games and activities geared to children. Find a farmers market near you at www.localharvest.org.

PARTICIPATE IN A COMMUNITY GARDEN   Most major metropolitan areas have community gardens, a designated green space parceled into sections to be rented and tended to by local community members. Community garden members each get a small plot of land for personal growing. Busy families often participate because members often help one another by tending to one another's gardens and sharing what's harvested.

SET UP A SCHOOL GARDEN   The National Farm to School Network (www.farmtoschool.org) offers many free resources online to help students, their families, and school staff create farm-to-school programming. Whether you create a school garden or connect with a local farm to support their efforts, the benefits of these programs are backed by extensive research. Start by getting together a group of parents or students who are interested in farming, eating healthy, and/or gardening to establish group support and divide the responsibilities.

EAT FARM TO TABLE Also referred to as "Farm to Fork," this movement brings local food to consumers through neighborhood restaurants, cafes, school and hospital cafeterias, and more. Find these establishments by asking your local farmer for recommendations for restaurants that buy from them and other local producers. Or visit the online resource knowwhereyourfoodcomesfrom.com, which offers directories of local farm-to-table restaurants for most states in America.[9]

CREATE A VEGETABLE GARDEN You don't need a huge yard or a green thumb to have a vegetable garden nowadays. Growing your own produce is practically foolproof with the latest gardening contraptions. Choose the size and approach that's right for your family.

Use potted plants Using pots to grow your own vegetables, herbs, and some types of fruit is one of the simplest ways to begin connecting your family directly with your food source. Be sure to choose varieties that work best in containers—both online suppliers and local garden supply stores will have this information. Children can choose to grow anything from peas to cucumbers and even lemons, depending on your growing zone. Check the online USDA Plant Hardiness Zone map (www.planthardiness.ars.usda.gov) to find your zone.

Try an EarthBox This amazing contraption is container gardening at its best. According to the manufacturer, "It is self-watering, sustainable, movable, and can even be used to grow indoors."[10]

Grow inside If your family has a sunny window or sunroom, you can grow some delicious varieties of vegetables, fruits, and herbs indoors without a special grow light. Lemons, mandarin oranges, tomatoes, peppers, basil, thyme, and rosemary are a few examples of plants you can grow indoors.

Build a raised bed A popular approach to home gardening requires building a large square or rectangle wood box outside that can be filled with fresh soil for planting. Handy families can cut wood and build a box from scratch, but there are plenty of raised bed kits available containing precut cedar wood and tool-free setup. Raised beds cost more, but they are much easier for families to maintain than in-ground plots, because they drain well, the fresh soil is ideal for your chosen plants, and fewer weeds tend to grow.

In-ground garden If you're feeling a little more adventurous and have time on your hands, consider creating a traditional garden in your yard. You need to plant seeds or seedlings (also called transplants) where sun is plentiful (usually at least six hours per day), space is available, the soil is rich with nutrients or you can amend it, and water drains properly. A gardening project is a perfect family learning opportunity. Children are more apt to eat food they help grow, so let them choose vegetable varieties from a list of easy-to-grow options suitable for your growth zone. Next, let kids measure between plants, dig and plant the seeds or seedlings, and participate in regular maintenance including watering, adding beneficial nutrients, and pulling weeds.

BE A GOOD FRIEND

I got you to look after me, and you got
me to look after you, and that's why.

– JOHN STEINBECK, *Of Mice and Men*

A SIMPLE CONVERSATION WITH a good friend can be transformative: it has
the power to turn what started as a horrible day into a joyful one. True
friends enrich our lives, provide moral support through ups and downs,
instill confidence, lift us up, and bring us joy. Sharing life with others
brings more meaning to everyday experiences and provides us with a
deeper sense of purpose. With the comfort of close relationships we have
security, stability, and strength to reach success and forge ahead through
adversity.

You don't need an eighty-year-long study to prove friendships are critical,
but the Harvard Adult Development Study, one of the world's longest
studies, has shown that what keeps us happy and healthy throughout life
is not fame or money, but close relationships.[1] Without true friends and
social companionship, we may feel that life is not worth living. The study
findings were dramatic: people with the fewest social ties and lowest-
quality social relationships were more likely to experience adverse
health outcomes and twice as likely to die than those with strong social

connections.[2] Having strong relationships is also a good predictor of health. The Harvard study found people most satisfied with their relationships at age fifty were also in the best physical health at age eighty.[3]

Studies show that the presence of a close friend during stressful times can suppress levels of the stress hormone cortisol.[4] Many studies also find having positive social ties wards off mental health issues. Consider how the emotional support of a friend during hard times may have benefited you or your family. Supportive friendships can limit the toll hardship takes on our health and remind us we still have some control over our lives.

Further, strong social support can positively influence the adoption of healthy behaviors. In adolescence, having positive peer relationships makes one less likely to participate in risky behaviors, such as drugs and alcohol, and resort to violence. As adults, when we genuinely care for and nurture others—such as children, spouses, and friends—we are more likely to take better care of our own health as well, so we can live longer and participate in life together.

YOUR INFLUENCE AS A PARENT

Developing intimate friendships in childhood is important, given the critical role friendships play in social and personal identity, social support, and psychological well-being. And parents are instrumental in guiding children on how to make friends and maintain relationships. One study followed children ages five to ten and discovered those children whose mothers helped them learn how to manage their negative emotions were more likely to have positive friendships at age ten than peers whose mothers did not provide this support.

In the world of social media, the word "friend" has taken on a whole new meaning. People now acquire friends by the hundreds. But true friendship requires far more investment and nurturing than liking photos and posting comments online. Adults and children who continue to nurture friendships through shared moments, co-created memories, and live interactions can create deep relationships that withstand the test of time.

THE CHANGE
BUILD MEANINGFUL RELATIONSHIPS.

PATH TO CHANGE   Close relationships are invaluable. It takes time and effort to grow and deepen relationships. Consider the following strategies for helping your family build new or strengthen old relationships:

MAKE TIME FOR PLAY DATES   Though technology can help people stay connected more often, it will never replace in-person interactions. Spending quality time with friends or partners develops emotional intimacy and creates history and lasting memories that strengthen bonds. You may not be able to meet up with friends as often as before you had kids, but it's still important to prioritize this time together. Schedule monthly or quarterly dates with friends to keep relationships strong and nurtured. The same goes for children. Since parents often dictate the schedule outside of school, it's important to set aside time for your children to spend with friends, as well. Encourage older children to invite a friend or two over to your house. For younger children, reach out to the parents of your children's classmates and buddies so you can proactively schedule play dates.

SHOW APPRECIATION Doesn't it feel good when someone tells you they love you, sends a card for no reason, or texts just to say, "You're great"? Expressing gratitude to your friends and family strengthens your relationships and makes the other person feel more satisfied in the relationship, too. Teach your children how to appreciate others by making it a regular habit to tell your spouse and your kids how important they are to you and how grateful you are for their companionship.

WORK IT OUT Disagreements and conflict are a natural part of life. And relationships tend to get stronger when people learn how to disagree and still remain friends. Instead of stepping in to resolve conflicts for your children, give them the tools to work it out on their own. Four useful tools for moving through conflict include taking personal responsibility for your actions leading up to the conflict, listening to the emotions of others, finding common ground, and learning how to agree to disagree. Practice them in your own life so you can find comfort in teaching them to your family, too.

SHARE WITH OTHERS Sharing with friends deepens relationships. Teach children to enjoy sharing by regularly sharing your favorite things with them, such as food, trinkets, and books, and discuss how it feels for both of you. Find opportunities for you and your family to share with people you care about or want to get to know better. For example, share garden tools with trustworthy neighbors, or make extra portions of dinner and bring them to a friend's house. Encourage your children to swap books, toys, or clothes with friends, too.

WEED OUT NEGATIVITY Negative relationships can be taxing to your family's emotional and physical health. Take steps to eliminate toxic relationships in your own life first, and share honest but age-appropriate explanations with your family about relationships you choose to eliminate, and why. Talk with your family about the tenets of being a good friend and the importance of being respected in a friendship. Meet your children's friends and inquire about their friendships so you can identify any unhealthy relationships and help your child move past them.

BE GOOD HOSTS Learning how to be hospitable can make all the difference in whether friends and your children's friends want to visit. Create a welcoming environment for parents of your children's friends (and your own friends) by having simple snacks and drinks available, greeting them at the door, taking their coats, and seeing them out. Teach children how to make guests feel welcome by sharing belongings, being kind, and staying present instead of on technological devices during the visit.

USE TECHNOLOGY TO STAY CONNECTED The use of texting, messaging, and video chat can make it much easier to stay connected with friends, both far and near. Use technology to tell friends you are thinking of them or to keep them up to date on your life. Schedule regular video chats with friends and family who live far away to keep connections strong. Encourage your shy or introverted family members to use technology to make initial contact with new friends less stressful.

HELPING KIDS

MANAGE FRIENDSHIP SITUATIONS

USE THE FOLLOWING strategies to teach your family how to work through tricky situations to forge a much smoother path in building friendships:

SITUATION	GUIDANCE
Being in a new place (school, community center, church) where you don't know anyone	**MAKE CONVERSATION:** Make new friends by starting a conversation. Ask questions and offer some information about yourself. Wait for answers, and don't talk the entire time. Give someone a compliment to get the conversation started.
Friend doesn't like the same thing as you	**APPRECIATE DIFFERENCES:** Join a friend when trying new activities or gaining new experiences. Ask questions to show your interest.
Friend is being mean or using mean words toward you or others	**SHARE YOUR FEELINGS:** It can be upsetting when a friend doesn't treat you nicely. Telling a friend how their actions make you feel may feel vulnerable, but it gives your friend a reason to change his or her ways. Take responsibility for your own actions as well.
Friends won't let you join in a game or activity	**BE RESOURCEFUL:** This will pass. Tell others you'd love to join whenever they are ready, and then find something else to do.
Friend tries to take an object from you	**BE POLITE:** Tell your friend how you feel and that you were not done with the object. Acknowledge that you see they want the object and that you'll give it to them once you are done with it.
It's hard to make friends	**RECOGNIZE POSSIBLE FRIENDS:** Connect with other children who share similar interests and values with you. Join in activities you enjoy to meet others with common interests. Practice how you might ask them to hang out outside of school or activities.

SMELL THE AROMA

The earth laughs in flowers.

—RALPH WALDO EMERSON

SCENTS HAVE POWERFUL effects on mood, memory, stress levels, and cognition. The smell of freshly baked banana bread may remind you of your grandmother's house, stimulating feelings of relaxation and contentment. The scent of freshly brewed coffee might instantly perk you up in advance of the caffeine. Scents can trigger specific memories and influence your emotions because your olfactory nerve, which is responsible for your sense of smell, is anatomically positioned close to areas of the brain that regulate emotion, emotional recall, and memory.

Essential oils derived from the flowers, leaves, stalks, and roots of plants have been used by many cultures for their physiological benefits. Aromatherapy is the practice of using scents from essential oils to intentionally shift emotions and improve well-being. Oils can be applied to skin by mixing them with carrier oils such as coconut or jojoba oil, or inhaled by using a room diffuser, a small electronic device similar to a humidifier.

Modern research has quantified the benefits of several commonly used oils, including lavender, bergamot, and orange. For instance, several studies show lavender oil helps children and parents get a good night's sleep.[1] Research has also shown lavender, bergamot, rosemary, orange, and cedarwood to be effective in managing stress and controlling anxiety symptoms.[2,3] One study found that children were less stressed and mentally anxious during dental procedures when orange essential oil was diffused in the room. Researchers measured a decrease in both pulse rate and salivary cortisol level.[4]

When used appropriately, essential oils are a safe and simple therapeutic tool that parents and children can use to promote joy, overcome sleep disturbances, or maintain emotional balance during stressful situations. And they can be used at any time, anywhere.

THE CHANGE
USE AROMATHERAPY TO PROMOTE RELAXATION, INCREASE ENERGY AND HAPPINESS, AND REDUCE STRESS.

PATH TO CHANGE   Use the following guidelines and tips to experiment with essential oils and safely incorporate them into your family's routines:

BUY PURE OILS; SKIP SYNTHETICS   The explosion of aromatherapy in the United States has resulted in a plethora of oil-based products available to consumers. The quality of essential oils, however, can vary greatly due to a number of factors in the growth and distillation processes. For example, harsh chemical solvents used by some manufacturers can negatively alter the health benefits of the oils. To find pure essential oils, choose a specialty retailer that is transparent about harvesting, distillation, and quality assurance. Trained aromatherapists prefer companies that test every batch of oil received from distillers to ensure authenticity. Testing results are typically included with the purchase of your oil or can be requested from the retailer.

BEWARE OF MARKETING LANGUAGE

There are no industry standards associated with quality of essential oils and no certifying organizations. As such, manufacturers and retailers are free to label their oils using any terminology. Companies often use a variety of terms to make their products sound superior. Don't be fooled by misleading claims. The following labels do not indicate superiority and do not have a standardized definition: *therapeutic, medicinal grade, clinical grade, and pharmaceutical grade.* Choose brands used by professional aromatherapists and/or companies that give consumers access to purity testing reports, called gas chromatography–mass spectrometry (GC-MS) reports.

AVOID PESTICIDES   Essential oils are highly concentrated. Producing an essential oil requires a large amount of plant matter; for example, three thousand organic roses are needed to make just .08 fluid ounce of NYR Organic's Rose Otto essential oil.[5] Therefore pesticides sprayed on plants will be more highly concentrated in an essential oil. To reduce your exposure to toxic pesticides, choose essential oils that are certified organic or unsprayed with pesticides.

HOW TO USE   Essential oils are typically inhaled or mixed with a carrier and applied to the skin (never apply undiluted oils directly to your skin). They should never be ingested, unless specific instructions appear on the bottle and the product is labeled as a dietary supplement, or formulated in a pill, tablet, or capsule. Use the following tips to experience the benefits of essential oils:

<u>*Vapor inhalation*</u>   Steam inhalation is a common method of aromatherapy. You can purchase a diffuser specifically designed to vaporize essential oils. To make a homemade version, add essential oils to boiling water to fill a room with a specific scent.

Baths and showers Add a few drops of essential oil to bath water or to the bottom of the tub before you run a shower. For instance, adding oils such as lavender and Roman chamomile can transform an ordinary bath into a relaxing oasis.

Massage oil or lotion Make your own personally scented massage oil or lotion by adding a few drops of essential oils to a gentle carrier oil such as virgin coconut oil, olive oil, or jojoba oil. Apply in small doses to specific areas of the body, or, for a larger impact, rub all over the body.

Compresses Essential oils can be beneficial for easing pain such as migraines or stomach cramps. To enjoy a compress, add a couple of drops of essential oils to a small bowl of warm or cool water, soak a washcloth and wring it out, and then apply to nonsensitive areas of the body. Avoid the eyes and pubic area.

Room spray For a quick and easy way to add aromatherapy to a room, create a personalized room spray. Combine 1 ounce alcohol, 2 ounces water, and 10 to 20 drops of your favorite essential oil in a small glass or metal spray bottle.

Insect repellent Some essential oils, such as geranium, thyme, mint, and patchouli, are used for their effectiveness in repelling insects.[6] Lemon eucalyptus has been studied and approved by the CDC as an effective mosquito and tick repellent, a more natural and safer option compared to DEET-based repellents. Try mixing a few essential oils to create your own homemade blend for repelling insects. Please note: When traveling abroad or to areas where insects (such as ticks) carry debilitating diseases such as Lyme disease, we recommend using a clinically proven and tested repellent instead of a homemade version.

ESSENTIAL OILS[7]

ESSENTIAL OILS CAN support health and improve a wide range of ailments. Choose favorite scents for common concerns.

OIL NAME	JOY	RELAXATION OR SLEEP	STRESS AND ANXIETY	ENERGY AND FOCUS
Basil				X
Bergamot	X	X	X	
Black pepper	X			X
Cedarwood		X	X	
Chamomile (Roman)	X	X	X	
Clary sage	X	X	X	
Frankincense		X	X	X
Geranium	X	X	X	
Ginger	X			
Grapefruit	X			X
Jasmine	X	X	X	X
Lavender	X	X	X	
Lemon				X
Lemon eucalyptus		X		
Mandarin	X	X	X	
Orange		X	X	
Patchouli	X	X	X	
Peppermint	X			X
Rose	X	X	X	
Rosemary	X		X	X
Sandalwood	X	X	X	
Ylang ylang	X	X	X	X

EXPLORE NATURE

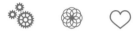

Look deep into nature, and then you will understand
everything better.

—ALBERT EINSTEIN

SPENDING TIME IN nature may be one of the best ways to boost family
health and happiness. Numerous studies show that adults with more
exposure to natural environments and green space have better mental
health and well-being, including less stress, anxiety and depression, and
significantly fewer cardiometabolic conditions.[1,2,3] In one study, participants were assigned to walk for fifty minutes in either a natural or an
urban setting. Psychological tests administered before and after the walk
found that participants assigned to a natural setting had experienced
improvements in working memory, as well as decreases in both anxiety
and excessive rumination over anxiety-provoking thoughts.[4]

Similarly, studies have shown that when children are immersed in
nature, they have enhanced mental and physical health, including
marked improvements in problem solving, mental cognition, patience,
and attention.[5] Natural environments can be especially helpful for
children suffering from attention deficit hyperactivity disorder (ADHD).
One study showed a three-fold decrease in symptoms with exposure to
natural environments.[6] Nature also promotes creativity and resilience.
For example, children are more imaginative and varied in their play

when they play in dirt or sand, or around trees and boulders, compared to when they play on human-designed playgrounds. Further, in natural settings, children encounter new experiences that test their resolve, and build their self-esteem and confidence.

DID YOU KNOW?

The amount of time children spend outside has declined dramatically over the past thirty-five years. According to the Institute for Social Research at the University of Michigan, in 1981 children spent an average of 140 minutes outside weekly versus only fifty minutes in 2003—a 180 percent decline![7] In 2011, a study of 8,950 preschoolers found children had an average of 4.1 hours of screen time daily (far more than other estimates of two hours daily), and only 50 percent of the children went outside with a parent to play each day.[8,9]

As a society, we are spending less time outdoors in nature than ever before. The Institute for Communications Technology Management indicates Americans spend twice as many hours consuming media each day as we did in 1960.[10] Families also spend a great deal of time shuttling between children's organized activities and little time on unstructured outside exploration. Further, urban sprawl has replaced former green spaces with residences and commercial property, thereby reducing access to natural environments. A growing body of research shows that the disconnection between nature and humans, especially in children, is associated with a decline in health. Richard Louv, author and founder of the Children and Nature Network, refers to this issue as "nature deficit disorder."

Families who participate in activities in the natural world can avoid this deficit and enhance their mental and physical well-being. Natural environments are free from television, wireless networks, and the hustle and bustle of everyday life, which allows families to slow down, connect, and explore together. And since observing nature exposes us to phenomena that are bigger than ourselves, time in nature supports spirituality and deepens our understanding of our world. Finally, regular exposure helps families develop an appreciation for nature and its importance to broader society. Children instinctively become environmentalists who protect the earth for the benefit of future generations.

DID YOU KNOW?

The Japanese practice a tradition called Shinrin-yoku, also know as forest bathing, where people take multiday trips to the forest for health benefits. Customary forest bathing has been studied extensively for its ability to lower cortisol levels, blood glucose, and blood pressure.[11]

THE CHANGE
PRIORITIZE TIME IN NATURE.

PATH TO CHANGE   Your family can enjoy the benefits of getting into nature, regardless of location or skill level. Nature-loving families can develop new skills by trying nature-based activities together, and nature newbies can start with easily accessible, equipment-free activities. Use the following tips to get started:

STROLL IN A NEIGHBORHOOD WITH TREES   If you live on a busy road or in a city, your family will reap more physiological benefits if you can walk through a neighborhood filled with trees and fewer cars. Population studies show that people living in areas with more tree cover have better mental and physical health.[12]

VISIT PARKS AND GREEN SPACE   Exploring America's public parks is one of the best ways for families to enjoy nature. There are thousands of state and national parks from which to choose, and cities have even begun prioritizing the creation and preservation of green spaces and greenways. Find a nearby park to visit regularly, or research the parks in your state so you can schedule trips to visit and explore them on weekends.

JOIN A LOCAL ENVIRONMENTAL GROUP Become members of a local chapter of the National Audubon Society or Sierra Club, not-for-profit organizations dedicated to wildlife and environmental conservation. Local chapters offer educational programming and events for adults and children that support efforts in conserving nearby wildlife and their natural habitats.

NATURE-BASED CAMPS AND SCHOOLS Summer camps offer children of all ages the opportunity to grow, develop, and learn in nature. Most nature-based camp programs now offer daytime sessions over summer months and school vacation weeks. Young children can also attend forest-based kindergarten or preschool programs (also called "classrooms without walls") for an age-appropriate, nature-based experience—find a nearby program at www.naturalstart.org. Or, as a family you can partici- pate in nature-based programming through classes offered by Tinkergarten—find a nearby class at www.tinkergarten.com.

GARDEN All family members can benefit from gardening. As a family, you can plant a flower garden or grow vegetables. Make gardening and yard work a regular family activity. For more guidance on gardening, see Week 15, Know Your Farmer.

GO CAMPING Sleeping in a tent or cabin gives families an opportunity to become completely immersed in nature. America has thousands of beautiful public campsites throughout the country located near lakes, beaches, forests, and mountains. When camping, your family can enjoy many nature-based activities such as birding, hiking, stargazing, animal tracking, and more. Find and reserve a local campsite on recreation.gov.

GET IN THE WATER Your family can soak up the beauty of nature at a lake, pond, or river or at the beach. Kayaking, canoeing, and stand-up paddleboarding are fun family activities, even for novices. You can rent all the equipment you need, right down to the life jackets. Plus, many equipment rental companies offer free lessons or guided experiences. Families with very young children can still enjoy natural water settings by choosing to swim or fish instead.

ENJOY OUTDOOR WINTER ACTIVITIES Most nature-based winter activities, such as cross-country skiing, snowshoeing, and sledding, require some type of equipment. But you can get started in all of these activities with very little training. Bundle up and immerse your family in the natural winter wonderland.

CHOOSE GRAINS WISELY

Nothing ventured, nothing gained, sometimes you've got to go against the grain.
—GARTH BROOKS

WHOLE GRAINS ARE the foundation of a healthy diet. But according to a 2015 survey by the Whole Grains Council, only 31 percent of Americans always choose whole grains over unhealthy refined grains.[1]

The health profile of a whole grain is vastly different from that of a refined grain. Whole grains contain three edible parts: the bran, the germ, and the endosperm. The bran is rich in fiber, B vitamins, antioxidants, and many minerals, including iron and zinc. The germ supplies healthy fats, vitamin E, B vitamins, and antioxidants. And the endosperm, the starchy center, contains very few nutrients except carbohydrates and some protein. Unlike whole grains, refined grains are stripped of the bran and germ parts during the manufacturing process, leaving only the endosperm, a stripped grain that lacks fiber or healthy fats and retains very few vitamins and minerals.

As you might realize, refined grains are no longer nutritious foods. Without the bran and germ layers to slow digestion, the starchy endosperm grain is quickly converted to glucose, causing blood sugar levels to spike and then drop rapidly—resulting in hunger and cravings for more sugar or refined grains. Some manufacturers try to boost the nutritive value of refined grain products by adding back lost nutrients, but these ingredients are often synthetic or partial components, and much less healthy than the original whole grain food.

DID YOU KNOW?

One of the many reasons whole grains are more healthful than refined grains is because they produce smaller fluctuations in blood sugar levels. Glycemic index is the measure, from 1 to 100, used to determine how quickly the body converts a carbohydrate-rich food into glucose—higher numbers indicate a more rapid and detrimental effect. See how whole grains stack up to refined grains:

GRAIN PRODUCT	GLYCEMIC INDEX[2]
Baguette, white, plain	95
Shredded wheat (Nabisco)	83
White wheat flour bread (average)	75
Whole wheat bread (average)	69
Whole grain bread (Conagra)	64
White rice (boiled, average)	64
Pumpernickel bread	56
Brown rice (boiled, USA)	50
Cracked wheat (bulgur)	46
Coarse barley bread, 80 percent kernels	34
Pearled barley (average)	25

You may have read recommendations to avoid any kind of grains. However, whole grains (particularly gluten-free versions) provide many health-promoting benefits, especially for growing children. For example, in an analysis of over 700,000 people, researchers found that those who ate four servings of whole grains daily (~70 grams/day) had about a 20 percent lower risk of death from both cardiovascular disease and cancer compared to people who ate little or no whole grains.[3] Replacing refined grains with whole grains also reduces your family's risk of diabetes, a growing concern even for children. In another study, researchers who assessed the dietary and health habits of over 161,000 women for a period of twelve to eighteen years found that every two servings of whole grains consumed per day was associated with a 21 percent decrease in the risk of type 2 diabetes.[4] Finally, fiber-rich whole grains improve digestive health, which is vital to a strong immune system. Up to 20 percent of the population suffers from chronic constipation;[5] consuming more whole grains bulks up stool, making it easier to pass, eliminating toxins, and boosting immune function.

THE CHANGE
REPLACE REFINED GRAINS WITH WHOLE GRAINS.

PATH TO CHANGE   Crowd out unhealthy refined grains and instead feed your family nutritious whole grains.

GET TO KNOW YOUR GRAINS There are so many whole grains to explore, your family will never get bored with the options.

GRAIN	FLAVOR/ TEXTURE	TIME TO COOK	SIDE/ SALAD	SOUP/ STEW	HOT CEREAL
Amaranth	Earthy, nutty, slightly sticky	30 min	X		
Barley* (pearled or hulled)	Slightly nutty, hearty, chewy	60 to 90 min	X	X	
Brown rice	Slightly sweet, sticky, firm	45 to 60 min	X	X	
Buckwheat (kasha) groats	Nutty, toasted, hearty	20 to 30 min		X	X
Bulgur* (cracked wheat)	Wheat taste, with light and airy texture	20 min	X		
Cornmeal (polenta)	Sweet, silky, yet slightly gritty	20 min	X		
Farro*	Like barley, but nuttier and sturdier	40 min	X	X	
Kamut*	Buttery, slightly sweet, soft like grits	90 min			X
Millet	Mild, sweet, fluffy, light	30 min	X		X
Oat groats	Nutty, sweet, chewier than oatmeal	75 to 90 min			X
Oatmeal (rolled/steel-cut oats)	Sweet, soft, smooth	20 to 30 min			X
Quinoa (keen-wah)	Mild, slightly nutty, firm	15 min	X	X	X
Rye berries*	Deep, hearty, nutty flavor	45 min	X		

GRAIN	FLAVOR/ TEXTURE	TIME TO COOK	SIDE/ SALAD	SOUP/ STEW	HOT CEREAL
Sorghum	Mild, earthy flavor much like wheat	60 min	X	X	
Spelt*	Like wheat but slightly milder and softer	2 hours	X	X	X
Teff	Earthy, nutty	15 to 20 min	X	X	X
Triticale berries*	Similar in flavor and texture to a rye and wheat blend	40 to 50 min	X	X	X
Wheat berries*	Slightly earthy, nutty, hearty	60 min	X	X	X
Wild rice	Intensely earthy, firm	60 min	X	X	

*Contains gluten

UPGRADE TO WHOLE GRAINS   Adjust taste buds to whole grains by making modifications slowly. Start with the biggest offenders. For example, if pasta is a regular at your dinner table, engage your family in a taste test to find a new 100 percent whole grain pasta option.

Breakfast   Since it's common to eat refined grains at breakfast (such as in cereal and bread products), making a swap offers big benefits. Try steel-cut oats, rolled oats, buckwheat groats, quinoa porridge, low-sugar oat-based granola, and muesli. Make delicious overnight steel-cut oats by adding fruit and cinnamon to recommended grain/water ratio. Or turn quinoa into porridge by mixing with coconut milk, cinnamon, and a drizzle of maple syrup. If you choose to purchase flavored grain-based breakfast options, be sure to check the ingredients to avoid added sweeteners and unhealthy additives.

Bread   Most bread in the United States is made with refined grains or flour. "Whole wheat bread" does not mean _all_ the flour is whole grain.

Look for breads and tortillas marked with the 100 percent whole grain stamp. If you're buying bread from a local bakery, search the ingredients to find options containing only whole grain flour. "Wheat flour," "unbleached flour," and "enriched flour" are not whole grain.

Crackers   Unfortunately, children's snack crackers, such as Goldfish and wheat crackers, are among the biggest culprits for containing nutrition-poor refined forms of grain. In the past few years, many new cracker brands have emerged that produce whole grain versions, such as Mary's Gone Crackers, Doctor Kracker, and more. Since truly whole grain crackers are hearty and nutritious, families can consider them a key part of the daily diet instead of an unhealthy snack.

Pasta   Fortunately, whole grain pasta is not hard to come by now. Many traditional brands, such as Barilla and private label grocery store brands, now offer whole grain options. Whole grain pasta is denser and chewier than white pasta, and every brand tastes and cooks differently. Try different brands and cooking times to find your family's favorite.

Baking at home   Baking can be trickier than cooking when it comes to replacing refined flours with whole grain flours. Whole grain flours are denser than white flours. You can start by substituting half of the white flour with whole grain flour for cookies, muffins, quick breads, and pancakes. You will get the best results when using a recipe created specifically for using whole grain flours. Check out cookbooks and recipes online that use whole grain and alternative flours (such as coconut and almond flours).

FIND WHOLE GRAIN PRODUCTS   Until the Food and Drug Administration (FDA) issues a statement defining whole grains, manufacturers are free to define whole grains as they choose on packaging and in marketing materials. Use the following tips to find genuine, 100 percent whole grain products:

Whole grain stamps[6]   In 2017, the Whole Grain Council updated their stamps to help consumers find whole grain products more easily.

GOOD	BETTER	BEST
WHOLE GRAIN 20g or more per serving — EAT 48g OR MORE OF WHOLE GRAIN DAILY	**50%+** **WHOLE GRAIN** 32g or more per serving — 50% OR MORE OF THE GRAIN IS WHOLE GRAIN	**100%** **WHOLE GRAIN** 23g or more per serving — 100% OF THE GRAIN IS WHOLE GRAIN
At least 8 grams of whole grains per serving, but more than 50 percent of the grains not whole	At least 50 percent of whole grains that contain at least 8 grams of whole grains per serving	Made with 100 percent whole grains and contains 16 grams of whole grains per serving

Read labels   If you can't find the whole grain stamp on a package, check the ingredient list. A product containing whole grains should list either whole grains or _whole grain flour_, such as _whole grain millet flour_ or _whole grain wheat flour_. Conversely, if the ingredients include just flour or enriched flour of any type, you can be certain the grains have been refined and the nutritious parts have been removed.

Still unsure? Contact the manufacturer   Fortunately, social media such as Facebook and Twitter have made it much easier for consumers to connect with manufacturers of food products. Post a message to the company on your favorite social media platform to find out how many whole grains are contained in their product.

CONSIDER GLUTEN-FREE   Until recently, research focused primarily on its impact to digestive health in people with celiac disease or NCGS. But, in 2016, scientists showed that a family of nongluten proteins in wheat called amylase-trypsin inhibitors (ATIs) triggers immune reactions not just in the gut, but also throughout the body. This can worsen symp-toms for those with inflammatory conditions such as multiple sclerosis, asthma, and rheumatoid arthritis, amongst others.[12,13,14] If anyone in your family has an inflammatory condition, choose gluten-free whole grains only. Wheat and gluten-containing whole grains have the highest concen-trations of ATIs by far, but they are found in some other foods. Work with a qualified functional nutritionist to discover what foods beyond wheat and gluten may trigger your symptoms.

HEAL WITH TOUCH

> When you touch a body, you touch the whole
> person, the intellect, the spirit, and the emotions.
> —JANE HARRINGTON

THE SQUEEZE OF a hug, a pat on the back, and a gentle touch on the arm all warm your heart, but also induce powerful effects on your brain. The importance of touch starts at birth: for infants, adequate touch and sensory stimulation is critical for proper growth and cognitive development. Many studies show that preterm infants who receive touch therapy, such as infant massage or kangaroo care (when an infant is held skin to skin by caregivers) experience healthy weight gain more rapidly, score higher on mental and motor assessments, and have reduced incidence of neurological impairments.[1] As children grow, regular touch improves proprioception—the ability to sense one's own body and have spatial awareness of where one is. For children with autism, therapeutic massage has been shown to improve a child's behavior, self-regulation, and ability to be receptive to another person, including making eye contact, giving face-to-face attention, and listening.[2]

Massage is a safe and gentle therapy that can reduce anxiety, boost mood, lessen pain, and improve sleep.[3,4] Physiologically, massage relieves stress in several ways. A research review of several studies showed massage therapy lowered the stress hormone cortisol by an average of 31 percent, raised dopamine by an average of 31 percent, and increased serotonin by an average of 28 percent. Dopamine and serotonin are neurotransmitters responsible for the regulation of mood, satisfaction, and self-esteem.

HUG THERAPY

You don't need a professional massage to benefit from touch therapy—a simple hug or two has been shown to produce similarly powerful effects that boost happiness, lower stress, improve blood pressure, strengthen the immune system, and deepen bonds with others. According to touch researcher Tiffany Field, hugging stimulates the vagus nerve, thereby triggering a rise in oxytocin, a neurotransmitter studied for its role in lowering blood pressure, heart rate, and cortisol, while improving response to pain.[5,6] In one study of fifty-nine women, researchers found those who reported greater frequency of hugs from their partner were found to have higher levels of oxytocin at the start of the study, and greater reductions in increased heart rate and blood pressure after they experienced a stress-promoting activity.[7]

Even when words aren't spoken, the use of touch can strengthen relationships and break down barriers between individuals. Teaching children what is safe and healthy touching at home allows children to flourish emotionally and helps them differentiate between positive touch and undesirable touching. Touch conveys love, compassion, reassurance, and encouragement, thereby strengthening bonds with children. For example, in one study, mothers who applied massage to their babies had significantly higher rates of attachment than those who did not do baby massage.[8]

THE CHANGE
BRING TOUCH INTO DAILY FAMILY INTERACTIONS.

PATH TO CHANGE Increasing physical contact between family members can improve the emotional and physical health of the entire family:

HUG MORE Your family may be used to hugging in the morning or
before bed, but there's nothing like a random hug from someone you love
during the day. Find ways to incorporate hugs more naturally, such as
when you first see your spouse after work or when a child arrives home
from school. If you aren't typically an affectionate family, change the
dynamic by asking for more hugs. Your family members are sure to reciprocate the affection after it becomes a regular behavior.

HOLD HANDS Regardless of age, grab your child's hand during intense
parts of movies, or hold hands during a walk in the park. Hold hands
with your partner or spouse, too. If your teens aren't interested in holding
hands, link arms or walk with your arm around their shoulders.

MASSAGE EACH OTHER Incorporating massage into bedtime routines
helps family members wind down, while also increasing bonds. Opt
for medium-touch massage for improved sleep. According to research
studies, people who received medium-touch massage versus light-touch

massage experienced a bigger decrease in cortisol, higher levels of oxytocin, and increased white blood cell counts.[10] Though children may not be quick to reciprocate a massage, your partner may be. Offer to give each other timed massages as a way to connect and relax together at the end of the week. Take a class to learn various massage strokes to provide a more relaxing and effective experience for the person massaged.

GET PROFESSIONAL MASSAGES FOR PARENTS AND TEENS   As long as teens receive a signed letter of parental consent, it is perfectly legal and safe for your teen to get a professional massage. By scheduling a couples massage, both of you can be in the same room when getting a massage. Teens who participate in sports, dance, and other physically demanding activities will benefit greatly from therapeutic massage to relieve tension, loosen muscles, and relax.

INCREASE TOUCH THROUGH GAMES   Gentle touch can provide positive benefits as well. Find fun ways to incorporate more touch with your family using the following fun games:

<u>Back drawing</u> Like Pictionary, draw pictures or words on your child's back with your fingers. Younger children will love guessing what you draw.

<u>Piggyback rides</u> If your back allows, hoist your younger children up on your back for a little ride around the room. You'll stimulate giggles and provide an opportunity for natural connection.

<u>Roly-poly on the bed</u> Wrap your arms and legs around younger children and roll along the bed. Be sure to support yourself with hands and knees when you roll on top so you don't squish your little one!

LAP READING   Encourage younger children to sit on your lap when reading books together. In this position, you can give them a loving hug more easily. For older children who might be too heavy for your lap, sit with them between your legs or lie close together when reading.

DISCOVER YOUR TRUE NORTH

Try not to become a man of success,
but rather try to become a man of value.
— ALBERT EINSTEIN

VALUES ARE AT the center of everything you think and do. They represent your priorities and are the driving force behind who you are and what you stand for. Your values are a result of all of your experiences and influences throughout your lifetime, including your upbringing, your education, your religious affiliation, friends and family, and more. They are what you believe to be of utmost importance in your life and are essential to making decisions predicated on your best interest.

YOUR INFLUENCE AS A PARENT

Parental behaviors and actions strongly influence how children prioritize values in their own lives. In a national survey conducted by researchers at Harvard's Making Caring Common Project, 80 percent of youth respondents reported that their parents valued achievement and happiness over caring for others. Yet their parents reported that raising caring children was a top priority for them. Authors of the study suggest the disparity is likely because parental messaging and actions are in conflict with their beliefs. Parents may not realize that celebrating achievement more than other values—such as caring for others, cooperation, and kindness—may be sending a confusing message.[1] To avoid such confusion or misperceptions, parents will want to ensure that their actions and messaging are consistent with their values.

———————

Your values are not a result of your reactions or situation. They run deep and are fairly stable. They are the basis of your character, from which you can solve problems, find purpose, maximize opportunities, and continually grow. People who understand and live by their values are more confident in where they are headed and what they prioritize in life. In a world of vast and varied opportunities and choices, values help give us direction.

Psychologists find children learn about values through social observation and imitation. It's not until children enter the teenage years that they begin to consciously evaluate the values passed down by their families and begin shifting toward a more personalized set of values.

Although your values are highly specific to you as an individual, you can also identify family values, which guide you and your family together as a collective. And, of course, you can help your children identify their personal values, so they can benefit from knowing them as well.

THE CHANGE
CONSCIOUSLY MODEL YOUR PERSONAL AND FAMILY VALUES.

PATH TO CHANGE Family members will face difficult decisions and challenges that test their personal beliefs. Understanding your values will make your choices easier and cause less emotional strife. Use the following strategies to solidify your values as individuals and as a family:

A STRONG SENSE OF VALUES

DEFINING AND HAVING a strong sense of values provides a multitude of benefits.

+ **GOAL SETTING:** Following a life predicated on your values gives you direction in setting your goals. This enables you to set goals true to what is important to you, rather than what is important to others.

+ **BETTER DECISION MAKING:** Your values give you a foundation from which to make all decisions. They ensure that your actions are in alignment with what you find important. Without a solid understanding of your values, it is easy to base decisions on circumstances and social pressures, instead of on what you value.

+ **IT ENABLES HAPPINESS:** When we are clear on our values and make choices in alignment with them, we promote happiness. When we don't, we can experience internal conflict, which ultimately leads to discontent.

+ **IT BUILDS SELF-CONFIDENCE:** Staying true to your values helps build self-confidence. You feel surer of your choices, the decisions you make, your character, and who you are. Further, your behaviors are more consistent and authentic.

VALUES EXPLORATION   You probably can recite several personal values you find important, such as honesty, education, or love. And although values may shift over time, depending on your life stage, transformative experiences, and personal priorities, there are generally a few that are steadfast. Knowing the things you value most is important for each member of the family and as a collective unit. Start this journey by using the Explore Your Values worksheet in Part III: Tools and Resources to discover your values. When it comes to family values, have a discussion with your partner or spouse to identify them together so you can present them in a unified manner to the rest of the family.

IDENTIFYING THE TOP THREE   We may hold several values as highly important, but when it comes to modeling values consistently, it is helpful to narrow them down to three of your most important. Doing so will help you and your family prioritize and make decisions more easily. For personal values, ask yourself:

Which values feel most like me and represent aspects of what I genuinely cherish?

Which values do I act upon consistently?

What am I willing to fight for and make sacrifices for?

For family values, answer these questions together so that you all have a unified belief in what is important to you as a family.

DID YOU KNOW?

Though dynamics differ across American families, one study finds that parents prioritize many of the same values. According to a report by the Pew Research Center, parents view *responsibility* and *hard work* as the top two values to teach children. Other values that top the list include good manners, helping others, independence, and persistence.[2]

DIALOGUE VERSUS DISCOURSE   Be explicit with your family about what is most important in life. Talk openly about your family values, and engage in discussion about what each value means to each of you. Young children learn best through play, so role-play moral dilemmas and value-based living using their favorite toys, such as dolls or superheroes. For older children, ask their advice about your own moral dilemmas, and use the conversation both as a means to learn about what they value and as a teaching opportunity.

ACTIONS SPEAK LOUDER   Teaching your children values through words may not be as effective as demonstrating them. For example, telling your family to value generosity may land on deaf ears, whereas by engaging the family in collecting food, toys, or clothing to donate, you model that generosity is important. Children are highly perceptive and pick up on our actions and what they mean. After identifying the values you hope to teach your children, pair them with potential actions you can take to demonstrate and model those values.

FIND GOOD ROLE MODELS   Choosing the people who surround your immediate family on a regular basis can help reinforce values. Consider the values modeled by your children's teachers, caregivers, and coaches, and their friends' parents. When you see similarities, open a dialogue with these adults to discuss values they prioritize and how these translate (or not) into interactions with your children. Be curious and ask questions. You might be inspired by what you learn.

DISPLAY THEM PROUDLY   Display décor and wall art that speaks to family values. You can find a variety of prefabricated, framed art in home décor retailers, such as Pier One Imports, HomeGoods, Pottery Barn, and Ikea. For a more custom or handmade piece, shop at Etsy.com, an online marketplace focused on handmade and vintage items. Other ways to display your values include writing them on a chalkboard or whiteboard or spelling them out with magnetic letters on the refrigerator.

HELP YOUR FAMILY LIVE THEIR VALUES When family members demonstrate an interest in exploring or expressing a value, help and support them. For example, if your child loves animals and expresses interest in the value of community, bring her to a shelter where she can donate food and toys to dogs and cats, as well as give them attention and affection. If your child is interested in demonstrating the value of courage, talk with him about professions, activities, or experiences that exemplify this value. Similarly, if you and your spouse aren't living your values, shift priorities to give yourselves space and time to do so. Doing things that are in concert with your values will bring you happiness and fulfillment.

VALUE-BASED DISCUSSIONS There is great overlap between our values and current events, politics, faith, spirituality, and culture. Instead of avoiding conversations that bring on heavy, passionate discussion, use them as an opportunity to connect with your family. For example, openly discuss the candidates running for office and what you perceive to be their values. Talk with children about the injustices of the world and ask questions that get them thinking about how these events could affect them now or in the future. Think out loud when reviewing the current events news feed on your phone—it's a perfect way to engage curious minds.

SAMPLE VALUES LIST

REVIEW THE FOLLOWING list of values with your family to discover which ones align with your personal beliefs. Although not an exhaustive list, it's good inspiration.

Acceptance	Determination	Independence	Reverence
Accomplishment	Development	Individuality	Risk taking
Accountability	Devotion	Innovation	Selflessness
Accuracy	Dignity	Insightfulness	Self-reliance
Achievement	Discipline	Inspiration	Sensitivity
Adaptability	Discovery	Integrity	Serenity
Adventure	Drive	Intelligence	Sharing
Altruism	Effectiveness	Intensity	Significance
Ambition	Efficiency	Intuition	Silence
Amusement	Empathy	Joy	Simplicity
Assertiveness	Empowerment	Justice	Sincerity
Attentiveness	Endurance	Kindness	Skill
Awareness	Energy	Knowledge	Solitude
Balance	Enjoyment	Leadership	Spirit
Boldness	Enthusiasm	Learning	Spontaneity
Bravery	Equality	Liberty	Stability
Brilliance	Ethics	Logic	Status
Calm	Excellence	Love	Stewardship
Candor	Experience	Loyalty	Strength
Capability	Exploration	Mastery	Structure
Careful	Fairness	Maturity	Success
Challenge	Family	Moderation	Support
Charity	Fearlessness	Motivation	Surprise
Clarity	Feelings	Openness	Sustainability
Cleanliness	Ferociousness	Optimism	Talent
Commitment	Fidelity	Order	Teamwork
Common sense	Focus	Originality	Thankfulness
Communication	Fortitude	Passion	Thoroughness
Community	Freedom	Patience	Thoughtfulness
Compassion	Friendship	Peace	Tolerance
Concentration	Fun	Performance	Toughness
Confidence	Generosity	Persistence	Tradition
Connection	Goodness	Playfulness	Tranquility
Consciousness	Grace	Poise	Transparency
Consistency	Gratitude	Potential	Trust
Contentment	Greatness	Power	Truth
Contribution	Growth	Productivity	Understanding
Control	Happiness	Professionalism	Uniqueness
Cooperation	Hard work	Prosperity	Unity
Country	Harmony	Purpose	Valor
Courage	Health	Quality	Victory
Courtesy	Honesty	Reason	Vigor
Creativity	Honor	Recognition	Vitality
Credibility	Hope	Reflection	Wealth
Curiosity	Humility	Respect	Welcome
Dedication	Imagination	Responsibility	Winning
Dependability	Improvement	Restraint	Zeal

TURN ON THE TUNES

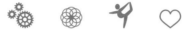

Music has healing power. It has the ability to take
people out of themselves for a few hours.

—ELTON JOHN

MUSIC IS INFUSED in all aspects of our culture—bringing us joy, invoking memories, and shifting our experiences. Music has the power to ignite emotion in all of us at every age; it can move us to dance, run, cry, or relax. It is a universal language that is beneficial to our health and well-being.

For starters, music can be used to lower stress and anxiety. A Cochrane review of twenty-three randomized controlled trials found listening to pre-recorded music had a moderate effect on reducing heart rate, blood pressure, and anxiety symptoms in patients with coronary heart disease.[1] While the stress-relieving benefits of music can be attributed in part to the distraction it provides, science shows that listening to music reduces inflammation while increasing expression of opiate receptors in your blood, both of which result in a calming effect.[2]

Music also stimulates parts of the brain associated with memory and cognitive function. It is believed that music helps us organize our thoughts, calms our spirit, and focuses our attention. For example, in a study of older adults, listening to classical music while doing other tasks improved episodic memory and processing speed over doing tasks in silence or with white noise.[3]

In children, listening to music has been shown to improve speech and language comprehension. In one study, nine-month-old infants participated in multimodal repetitive play sessions, either with music (such as waltzes) or without music. After just four weeks and a total of twelve sessions, researchers found that the infants exposed to the musical interventions had enhanced neural processing of both music and speech.[4] For these reasons language immersion programs for adults and children often use music and song to introduce new words and memorize them more quickly than conventional listen-and-repeat teaching methods.

Studies also show that enjoying music can have a positive impact on families as early as conception. Dr. Van Carr, a researcher, found that when parents played music for the baby in utero, the babies experienced significant benefits in areas of early speech, physical growth, parent-infant bonding, and success in breastfeeding, compared to those children and parents who did not provide musical stimulation.[5] As children grow, they and their parents can continue to enjoy music together to improve mood, deepen experiences, and bring more joy to life.

DID YOU KNOW?

It's never too late to benefit from musical training. A study of older adults between the ages of sixty-five and eighty years who received individualized piano instruction experienced enhanced executive function and memory compared to peers who did not receive piano lessons.[6] If you've always wished you could play the guitar or some other instrument, it's never too late to start private or family lessons to reap the benefits.

THE CHANGE
INCORPORATE MUSIC INTO FAMILY LIFE.

PATH TO CHANGE   Infuse music into everyday family life to bring more joy to otherwise typical activities. Some tips include:

CREATE A MUSIC LIBRARY   Choose a digital music platform with good search capabilities and premade playlists, so you can easily find the music you want, but also broaden your listening options.

INTERNET RADIO   Pandora and other internet radio providers offer apps for mobile devices and tablets, as well. Free access includes advertisements similar to typical radio stations, but you can upgrade your subscription to have ad-free listening. Unlike typical radio stations, you can "like" or "dislike" what is played to make the apps smarter and improve song selection.

Digital music service   Amazon Music, iTunes, Spotify, and other platforms give members access to millions of songs, curated playlists, and ad-free listening. Access varies by service, but most allow members to listen via apps on mobile devices, tablets, computers, and other devices.

Personal music library   Organize your music into a digital library on a home computer. Your whole family can connect to the library via smartphone apps and play music that suits their personal tastes and moods.

INCORPORATE MUSIC INTO EVERY DAY   Music can infuse joy and fun into everything from daily chores to Sunday barbecues. Think about how music can fit into your family's routine:

Daily meal prep/cleanup   Make cooking and cleaning more fun and enjoyable with energizing tunes such as Top 40, dance music, or jazz.

Music outdoors   Install a speaker system in your yard or on your porch or patio to enjoy music during gardening, grilling, and outdoor family gatherings. Keep the volume at a level that is considerate of your neighbors, too.

Commuting Personalize music in your car with satellite radio or a Bluetooth connection to a music app on your mobile phone. Rotate which family member chooses music so the whole family gets exposure to new genres.

ENJOY VARIETY   It's normal to favor one type of music, but there are greater benefits from enjoying a variety of genres. Researchers have discovered that different genres of music engage different areas of the brain. And people who listen to a variety of music engage both the auditory area of the brain and the emotional areas of the brain.[7] Keep your music library fresh, and explore different genres of music to provide even more brain-boosting benefits to your family.

KIDS LIKE QUALITY MUSIC   If you have young children it is very easy to get sucked into the routine of listening to kid-friendly tunes. Resist the temptation to placate them with repetitive, monotone songs. Children benefit from exposure to a variety of professional, high-quality musical genres to experience the cognitive benefits that music offers. Share classical, jazz, and popular modern music without explicit lyrics. For kid-friendly pop music, find the song on an album by Kidz Bop, an organization that records kid-friendly versions of modern Top 40 music (www.kidzbop.com).

USE MUSIC TO SHIFT EMOTIONS   Music has the power to shift moods and provide emotional support to your family. Play calming music to induce relaxation and soothe frazzled nerves. Listen to classical music during schoolwork or creative tasks. Incorporate upbeat music to increase energy levels and bring a quick boost of vitality into your home. And talk with children about how they can use music to support their personal emotional well-being.

MOVE TO THE MUSIC   Don't wait for a special event to celebrate with music. Spend time as a family singing, dancing, clapping, and moving to music to create joyful musical memories. According to Lilli Levinowitz, cofounder of Music Together, "children need to sing and move to the music to make meaning of it, a cognitive process called audiation."[8] Schedule those family dance parties!

SEE LIVE MUSIC   Watching and listening to musicians play live can transform your family from fair-weather music fans to music lovers. Seek out age-appropriate live music venues to share with your family:

The symphony   If you live near or in a city, look at local symphony and orchestra offerings. Many host family-friendly concerts.

Musicals   Traveling Broadway shows tour the country, making popular music productions available to almost all major metropolitan areas. Find out what is playing in your local city's playhouses.

Concerts   Children as young as nine years old can safely attend concerts with chaperones. Libraries will often host musicians. Be sure to review the music beforehand to ensure the tone of the concert will be age-appropriate. And hearing protection is essential.

MAKE MUSIC TOGETHER   Making music with your family offers profound benefits beyond just listening to music. According to Dr. Suzanne B. Hanser, author of *Manage Your Stress and Pain through Music,* "when you engage in active music making, you use more parts of your brain, exercise more parts of your body, and have a much more robust experience, particularly if you are improvising, creating something new, or harmonizing a melody."[9] Purchase kid-friendly musical instruments for younger children, and play simple tunes with them, such as "Happy Birthday" and "Twinkle, Twinkle, Little Star." For older children, consider buying used instruments or borrowing from the library. Watch YouTube videos or purchase professional lessons for the whole family to learn how to play instruments so you can play music together.

BE A CONSCIOUS CARNIVORE

If a kid ever realized what was involved in factory
farming, they would never touch meat again.

—JAMES CROMWELL

WHETHER YOU ARE an animal lover or not, the meat you eat, and where
it is sourced from, has a tremendous impact on your health. In America, the majority of animal products come from factory farms or animal
feeding operations (AFOs), defined by the EPA as "agricultural operations
where animals are kept and raised in confined situations."[1] For instance,
the majority of domestically produced pork comes from swine operations
housing over ten thousand hogs.[2] Since AFOs operate on disproportion-
ately small areas of land, animals must be confined in metal cages that
provide minimal opportunity for normal behavior, such as roaming and
grazing open land. Instead, they eat animal feed formulated to promote rapid growth at the lowest possible cost. Further, it often contains
antibiotics, arsenical drugs, animal byproducts, and other harmful
ingredients.[3,4] What's more, hormones and antibiotics are routinely
administered, chiefly to fatten the animals, but also to treat infections
that arise from the animals' eating unnatural food sources (such as cows
eating grain-based feeds instead of grass) and to prevent infections that
result from overcrowding and exposure to dead animals and excrement.

Eating meat and other animal products sourced from factory farms exposes your family to a variety of health risks. A review by the European Commission found increased risk of breast cancer and DNA damage associated with exposure to the hormones found in bovine meat and meat products—the review, conducted in 1999 and again in 2002, led to banning most American-produced bovine meat products in Europe.[5] A growing body of research also shows human exposure to low doses of antibiotics, such as the subtherapeutic amounts given to industrially raised animals, alters gut bacteria, and can cause weight gain and obesity.[6]

In many cases, the nutritional profile of industrial meat is poorer than its pasture-raised counterpart. This is likely due to lack of adequate exercise and the diminished nutrients in the industrial animal's unnatural food sources. Grass-fed steak has twice as many omega-3s and far less saturated fat than grain-fed steak. Pasture-raised meat may also be a safer choice for consumers, as research finds that open pasture chicken farms have significantly lower levels of salmonella and grass-fed cattle have far less E. coli.[7,8]

Fortunately, retail sales of sustainably raised meat and animal products are growing exponentially in the United States. Grass-fed beef sales have doubled anually, increasing from $17 million in 2012 to $262 million in 2016. By choosing sustainably raised animal products, your family will benefit from less exposure to toxic bacteria and unnecessary hormones, pesticides, and other chemicals. Given that the majority of meals are still eaten at home, families can protect and improve their health by simply upgrading the animal products consumed at home.[9]

DID YOU KNOW?

According to a 2010 report by Pew Charitable Trusts, just four corporations own the majority of U.S.-based livestock production, including beef (85 percent), chicken (51 percent), and pork (65 percent). Less competition causes prices to rise and eventually squeezes small and mid-size farmers out of the market.[10]

THE CHANGE
EAT ANIMAL PRODUCTS THAT DO NOT CONTAIN HORMONES, ANTIBIOTICS, CHEMICALS, AND OTHER HARMFUL, INDUSTRIALLY RAISED COMPONENTS.

PATH TO CHANGE Upgrade the animal products you eat:

UNDERSTAND LABELS Most labels used on animal products are not standardized, regulated, or verified. In some cases, even when a label is verified it does not ensure a better product. Both the Environmental Working Group and the Consumer Reports Food Safety and Sustainability Center conduct evaluations of food labels and provide clarifying information to consumers on their websites. For guidance, see "Deciphering Food Labels on Animal Products" on the following page.

ANIMAL PRODUCTS SERVED AT HOME It can be confusing to know the differences between animal products that are grass-fed, organic, or free-range. Refer to the following tips to find the best version of animal products to serve your family.

Milk and butter Avoid exposure to genetically engineered growth hormones (rbGH or rbST) injected in dairy cows by choosing milk and butter labeled either organic or American grass-fed, as both prohibit the use of growth hormones. Bonus—grass-fed dairy has higher levels of beneficial omega-3 fatty acids.

Cheese For domestically produced cheese, buy organic or American grass-fed to avoid exposure to growth hormones. Imported cheese from Europe or Canada is safe because growth hormones are banned.

Beef AFO cattle are injected with growth hormones and fed pesticide-ridden, grain-based feeds to fatten them up more quickly. Cows that eat grain instead of grass get sick more often and require antibiotics to

ON ANIMAL PRODUCTS

FOOD LABELS ON animal products can be highly confusing to even the most informed consumer. Use the table as a guide to which labels are meaningful and verified. Check Greener Choices (www .greenerchoices.org/labels/) for the most updated information.

| LABEL | REQUIREMENTS TO USE THE LABEL: | | ANTIBIOTICS AND GROWTH HORMONES PROHIBITED | DEFINITION |
	Application required?	*Verification process?*		
All-Natural or Naturally Raised	No	No	No	No common standard definition.
Animal Welfare Approved*	Yes	Yes, on-site farm inspection	Yes	Animals raised humanely on a family farm from birth to slaughter in well-managed pastures.
Cage-Free	No	No	No	No common standard definition. For chickens, this label is allowed but has *no meaning* because broilers are typically not raised in cages.
Free-Range	Yes, only for beef and poultry (not eggs)	No	No	Cattle must have outdoor access for 120 days of the year. Poultry must have some outdoor access. No requirements for the size or condition of outdoor space.

Sources: Consumer Reports Food Safety and Sustainability Center and Environmental Working Group

*Verified by USDA or Third-Party Agency

| LABEL | REQUIREMENTS TO USE THE LABEL: | | ANTIBIOTICS AND GROWTH HORMONES PROHIBITED | DEFINITION |
	Application required?	*Verification process?*		
Global Animal Partnership Steps 1 to 5+*	Yes	Yes, on-site inspection conducted by third party every 15 months	Yes, some hormones allowed in breeding	Animals raised on farms meet a set of animal welfare standards specific to the designated step. Step 1 has the fewest requirements; Step 5+ is the most animal-centered. Steps 4, 5, and 5+ are among the healthiest options.
No Added Hormones, *or* Raised Without Hormones, *or* No Hormones Administered	Yes, only for beef and sheep	No	Yes (for hormones); antibiotics or other substances allowed	No hormones are used, but breeder pigs are still allowed to receive hormones even when this label is applied to the offspring.
Pasture-Raised	No	No	No	No standard definition. Can be helpful when found on meat and poultry because USDA requires producers to include their definition on the package.
Raised Without Antibiotics	Yes, only for meat (not dairy or eggs)	No	Yes (for antibiotics), growth hormones allowed	For meat, no antibiotics are used. For dairy and eggs, USDA has no standard definition.
USDA Organic*	Yes	Yes, on-site inspection conducted by certified third party	Yes	Animals fed 100 percent organic certified feed, allowed year-round outdoor access, and raised on certified organic land.

stay alive. Choose certified grass-fed beef or organic beef (though the organic label does not prohibit feed from containing grains) to avoid exposure to hormones, antibiotics, and chemicals.

Pork Avoid exposure to growth hormones and antibiotics by choosing pork labeled organic or "Animal Welfare Approved." Growth hormones are illegal in pork production. Instead farmers routinely use ractopamine—a synthetic drug that promotes muscle growth and is banned in 160 countries, including China—and antibiotics for growth promotion.

Poultry The USDA prohibits growth hormones in poultry, so operators tend to overfeed and provide minimal space for movement in order to rapidly increase the chickens' size and weight. Laws require organic chickens to eat organic feed and have access to the outdoors (though space allowances are not regulated). For chicken that has been allowed to forage in a pasture, look for the "Animal Welfare Approved" label.

Eggs Laying hens are typically raised in caged housing systems that allow them to stand up but lack enough space for them to turn around or stretch their wings. Over 80 percent of the antibiotics produced in the United States are given to livestock and poultry, a process that contributes significantly to the growth of antibiotic-resistant bacteria. Choose eggs labeled "USDA Organic," "Animal Welfare Approved," or "Certified Humane." Eggs from hens raised on pastures have higher levels of healthful omega-3 fatty acids.

Fish See Week 31, Go Fish, for guidance on buying high-quality fish.

Deli meat and hot dogs Most hot dogs and deli meats come from factory-farmed animals but also contain unhealthy fillers and additives. Since children love these versions of meat, it is important to serve the healthiest versions by choosing organic and nitrate-free brands.

SERVE NONTRADITIONAL MEATS   Nontraditional meats are typically sourced from local hunters or smaller breeders. By choosing wild meat and milk, you can avoid exposure to chemicals and other toxic products common to industrial animal production.

Bison or buffalo Similar to beef, this red meat is much leaner and tastes slightly gamier. According to the National Bison Association, growth hormones and feed with synthetic components that artificially promote growth are prohibited.[11]

Ostrich Surprisingly, it tastes more like beef than like poultry.

Venison Deer meat, which tastes like beef, but with a gamier flavor.

Quail Has a stronger flavor than chicken or turkey, but is typically prepared similarly and enjoyed by many food enthusiasts.

Goat Goat cheese, milk, and yogurt have become widely available in the United States and are often produced on sustainable farms. Goat is traditionally eaten in developing countries such as India, Pakistan, Nepal, and Bangladesh, but has become increasingly popular in America.

SAVE MONEY; BUY THE WHOLE ANIMAL Sustainable meat is often much more expensive than factory-farmed meat. But by purchasing the entire animal from a local farmer, you'll pay less, because farmers save money on sales and marketing operations. When stored in a deep freezer, meat typically lasts for six months to a year. If this is too much meat for your family, share the purchase with other families!

EMBRACE FROZEN Unless otherwise specified, grocery stores feature industrially raised animal products in the meat department cases. Find organic or grass-fed meat in the freezer section. If slaughtered and immediately frozen, defrosted frozen meat can often taste much better than the fresh meat that sits in the meat cases for days.

EAT MORE VEGETARIAN PROTEINS, ESPECIALLY WHEN DINING OUT Like grocery stores, the majority of restaurants source industrially raised animal products unless otherwise specified. Choose restaurants that serve sustainably raised animal products, or order vegetarian dishes that feature beans or whole grains.

TOSS PLASTICS

Only we humans make waste that nature can't digest.
—CHARLES MOORE

PLASTIC IS PERVASIVE. In our modern society, it is virtually impossible to avoid it. Plastic is found in everything from car parts to appliances, food packaging to furniture. Without plastics, advancements in medical devices, technology, and consumer goods wouldn't exist. In her book *Plastic: A Toxic Love Story*, Susan Freinkel captures it well: "Plastics freed us from the confines of the natural world, from material constraints, and limited supplies that had long bounded human activity." Unfortunately, with time, science has found there is a price to pay for our deep-rooted reliance on plastics.

Images of birds caught in plastic rings and sea creatures wrapped in plastic bags convince us that plastics are bad for the environment. However, human exposure to the chemicals in plastic is even more troubling. When plastics break down over time, the chemicals released into food and beverages are absorbed into skin or released into the air, making them easily inhaled, which is harmful to our bodies. For example, extensive evidence shows bisphenol A (BPA), a chemical used to harden plastics, disrupts hormones and is linked to infertility, breast and reproductive system cancer, diabetes, early puberty, and behavioral changes in children.

Phthalates are another class of chemicals used as binding agents in plastic to make it flexible. Research shows that phthalates disrupt hormones and are linked to early onset of puberty in girls, and problems with male reproductive systems, including infertility, lower semen quality, and deformation of the testes.[1,2] Though some phthalates are banned in children's products, they persist in food packaging and consumer goods (such as shower curtains).

There's an effort to reduce plastic coast to coast, from cities banning the use of plastic bags to teens taking the lead to eliminate plastic waste in their schools. Families who participate in this nationwide charge against plastic are more likely to raise plastic-conscious children and reduce their family's long-term exposure to its toxic chemicals.

DID YOU KNOW?

BPA-Free isn't better for you. Due to the extensive evidence against BPA, manufacturers rushed to replace BPA in products with chemicals such as bisphenol S and F. But research shows that these replacements are not only similar in chemical structure but also have harmful endocrine-disrupting effects like their troublesome cousin, BPA.[3]

THE CHANGE
TOSS OUT PLASTICS.

PATH TO CHANGE   Reduce your family's exposure to toxic chemicals in plastics with the following tips:

UPGRADE FOOD AND WATER STORAGE CONTAINERS   Research shows plastic containers release estrogenic chemicals, or hormone disruptors, that mimic the actions of natural estrogen, especially after being exposed to common stressors. One study that tested over 450 commercially available plastic products found that the majority of all products, including BPA-free water and baby bottles, released estrogenic chemicals after being exposed to the microwave, boiling water, or UV light (that is, sunlight).[4] Swap out plastic for the following alternatives:

<u>Glass</u> Most glass food storage containers and baby bottles can be safely used in the refrigerator, freezer, oven, microwave oven, and dishwasher. Unlike plastic, glass is stable, so there is no risk of chemical leaching. Your family can also use glass water bottles, often covered in a silicone sleeve to avoid breakage, instead of BPA-free bottles.

<u>*Try stainless steel*</u> Many beverage and food containers and thermoses use stainless steel. When insulated, these containers provide the added benefit of keeping liquids hot or cold for extended periods of time. Use stainless steel containers for food storage and packing children's lunches.

<u>*Paper snack and sandwich bags*</u> Unbleached natural parchment paper is a great way to pack snacks and sandwiches. Even better, it's now available in bag form.

<u>*Reusable pouches*</u> Store snacks and sandwiches in reusable cloth pouches that come in a variety of sizes and patterns. Note that some reusable pouches are not made from cotton and may contain harmful chemicals, including phthalates, PVC, vinyl, or EVA. Check the ingredients, or search for 100 percent cotton bags that you can launder between uses.

AVOID PLASTIC WRAP AND PACKAGING When possible, purchase fresh food that isn't packaged in plastic. For example, opt for freshly picked bundles of spinach in lieu of plastic bags or containers of spinach. And avoid using plastic wrap to preserve food; instead, cover food with glass plates or use glass containers. If plastic packaging is unavoidable, lower your family's exposure to plastic chemicals by transferring food from plastic packaging to glass after purchase. According to Robin Whyatt, professor of environmental health sciences at the Columbia University Medical Center,

"DEHP in plastic continues to leech over time, so you reduce exposure by changing the storage container even if it was bought in plastic."[5]

CHOOSE CLOTH SHOWER CURTAINS PVC is the most toxic plastic chemical, yet many household products, including shower curtains, are made of it. Plastic shower curtains emit toxic chemicals over time, especially with exposure to hot water and steam.

TAKE PRECAUTIONS WITH TOYS AND CRAFTS Since infants and young children explore their world by putting toys (and everything else!) in their mouths, it is best to use silicone-based or wooden toys. Choose manufacturers who have explicitly committed to avoid the use of unhealthy, toxic ingredients, because they can often lurk in unexpected places. Even low-level exposure to the chemical asbestos has been shown to cause cancer and other fatal lung diseases.[6]

CLEANER COOKWARE Teflon, the plastic material used in nonstick pans, originally contained a hazardous carcinogen called C8. After huge fines to the manufacturer and lengthy legal battles, C8 was banned worldwide.[7] The chemicals that replace C8 in nonstick cookware are newer, and their safety is not well established. Avoid risk to your family by skipping nonstick and aluminum pans; instead use cookware of stainless steel, cast iron, or ceramic, a nontoxic alternative to nonstick.

AVOID BPA IN CANS As mentioned, BPA is an established endocrine-disrupting chemical, often found in the lining of food cans. Though many manufacturers have removed BPA from cans, most (except Eden Foods) are not forthright about which resins are used in place of BPA. Eden Foods uses Oleoresin in their BPA-Free cans, or a mixture of oil and substances from various plants. When in doubt, if your favorite canned food has BPA (or a healthier alternative such as that used by Eden Foods), opt instead for food stored in glass jars, or choose frozen.

HAVE REAL CONVERSATIONS

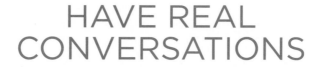

Everything becomes a little different
as soon as it is spoken out loud.
—HERMANN HESSE

HUMANS CRAVE CONNECTION, and the ability to converse enables us to develop and deepen the bonds we have with other people. Sherry Turkle, MIT communications professor and noted author, says, "Face to face conversation is the most human—and humanizing—thing we can do."

With the growth of text, tweeting, and posting online, having a real conversation may be on the decline. Turkle says, "The world is more talkative now, but it's at the expense of actual conversation." For example, some studies found young adults who attend college today are 40 percent less empathetic than generations before![1] Researchers believe that since current students are spending significantly more time communicating online rather than in face-to-face discussions, they are unable to effectively evaluate facial expressions to detect another person's emotions.

In the home, the proliferation of screens and wireless communications is putting the parent-child relationship at risk, as well. Meaningful conversation between parents and their children is extremely critical for development of a child's language skills, emotional intelligence, self-esteem, and ability to manage conflict. Further, research finds children's well-being is directly related to how often they talk with their parents about meaningful topics. In one research study, children with the highest well-being score reported having meaningful conversations with their parents every day.[2]

As children grow into adolescence, conversations between teenagers and their parents directly influence teen decision-making and risk-taking behavior. For example, it is well documented that teenagers who talk with their parents frequently about sexual topics are more likely to delay sexual activity, practice abstinence, and use contraception if they do become sexually active. In one large study administered across six Boston high schools, 32 percent of teenagers reported parental communication would help deter teen pregnancy, and of the 35 percent of teenagers using contraception, 49 percent talked with their parents frequently about sexual matters.[3] Another literature review found "teenagers make better sexual decisions when they have frequent and meaningful conversations with their parents, characterize the relationship with their parents as close, and feel their parents are comfortable and open when talking about sexual matters."[4]

Similarly, teens are less likely to smoke, drink, and use drugs when they have regular, open, and constructive discussions with their parents about real-life scenarios, peer pressure, and past parental experiences. Conversely, when parent-child conversations focused purely on rules around alcohol and drugs, teenagers were more likely to engage in these risky behaviors.[5,6]

Meaningful conversations need time to unfold, space for silence and reflection, and consistency to deepen. Creating an open dialogue with children is important to their well-being. In fact, one report by the Children's Aid Society found that children who did not feel free to express their ideas and opinions at home were six times more likely to report low well-being. It's time to join together, put down the screens, and rediscover the lost art of real conversation—for the sake of our happiness and the well-being of our family.

THE CHANGE
HAVE MEANINGFUL CONVERSATIONS WITH YOUR FAMILY EVERY DAY.

PATH TO CHANGE   Use the following strategies to have more meaningful discussions that deepen your familial relationships and establish lasting bonds:

TALK DAILY   Make it a priority to talk each day with every person in your family, including your partner or spouse, about topics that matter. Give yourself permission to ignore emails and let the dirty dishes sit overnight so you can engage in meaningful conversations.

Use the commute   Modern families are in the car *a lot*. Use this opportunity to share funny stories about your day, ask meaningful questions, or consider current events. When carpooling, be the parent who speaks and shows interest in your children and their friends.

Dinner conversation   Instead of cleaning the kitchen and prepping lunches, take time to sit with your family for a meal and undisturbed discussion. For people with attention problems, eating is a beneficial distraction that allows them to keep their hands busy and moving so they are better able to open up and connect.

Before bedtime Young children often process their day before falling asleep. Use bedtime as an opportunity to find out what is on your child's mind before turning out the lights. When children get older and become more independent with bedtime routines, resist the temptation to stay completely hands-off, and keep this time sacred for connecting about the day.

TAKE WALKS   Talking during long walks with your family is not only good for your relationship, but also good for your health.

REMOVE DISTRACTIONS   In a Pew Research Center report, 82 percent of American adults believe cell phone use in social gatherings hurts the conversation. Research finds that when smartphones are present, the conversations people have tend to focus on topics that do not require undivided attention. As Sherry Turkle put it, "Even silent phones disconnect us."[8,9] Consider implementing rules that restrict all media, homework, toys, and reading materials during conversation times, such as at mealtimes, bedtime, or family time.

BE A GOOD LISTENER   It is common for the person who talks the most in a conversation to also feel more positive and uplifted by that conversation. Practice active listening to be a good listener so you can deepen relationships. This is especially important when connecting with children, who are still developing the skills to formulate words to effectively express their feelings.

USE VERBAL JUDO   Getting your children to talk can feel like pulling teeth. But, according to child therapists, the answer lies within the questions we ask and the way in which we phrase our questions. First, instead of asking your child "How was your day?" ask questions that request more specific, interesting information, such as "What was the best part about your day?" or "Did someone do anything funny today?" You can also start a question with "I wonder whether. . ." Adding a few more words like these to our questions can make it feel less like an inquisition. Finally, try asking indirect questions to begin, such as, "If

Grandmother were to ask you, 'What are the five best things about being back at school?' what would you say?" If these strategies aren't working (especially with your teens and tweens), seek support from a professional to keep the lines of communication open in your family.

ASK FOR OPINIONS   Create conversation by sharing a personal situation of your own and requesting input from family members. You'll notice people of all ages feel proud and honored to offer their opinion, and you may even receive some helpful and interesting suggestions from your youngest children.

OPEN UP   Being in the company of people who are open and forthcoming about their experiences and feelings helps those who are timid or reserved feel more comfortable sharing their own feelings, too. Talk with your family about your own life, and resist keeping any topics off limits. When parents share their own experiences on topics such as drugs, alcohol, and sex, their teenagers begin to view them as more relatable and become more comfortable sharing in a similar fashion.

TAKE INTEREST IN THEIR INTERESTS   To create more opportunities for conversation with children, Adele Faber, author of *How to Talk So Kids Will Listen & Listen So Kids Will Talk*, recommends that parents take an active interest in children's passions, such as LEGOs, reading comic books, or playing music. Performing these activities together provides more opportunities for you to occasionally ask questions about other topics, too.

TALK IT OUT   After having an argument with a loved one, it's natural to want to take some time to cool off and let intense emotions fade. However, be sure not to skip reconciliation. While it certainly is easier to simply forget the situation and continue on with everyday life, it is especially important to make amends with children and find common ground. Learning how to make amends is an important skill for maintaining strong relationships. Extend the olive branch, as necessary, to initiate reconciliation with children, especially with stubborn tweens and teens.

NURTURE SPIRITUALITY

Spirituality is meant to take us beyond
our tribal identity into a domain
of awareness that is more universal.
—DEEPAK CHOPRA

IN JUST THE past decade, the number of Americans who do not identify
with any religion has grown by 50 percent, to include almost fifty million people.[1,2] Although religious affiliation is on the decline, Americans,
more than ever before, are defining themselves as "spiritual, but not
religious." Many religious people see spirituality and religion as one and
the same, but the growing population of unaffiliated spiritual individuals
views things differently. Spirituality is the belief that everything in this
universe is connected by some greater phenomenon that is bigger than
oneself—and the terms we use to describe this include "a higher power,"
"the universe," "nature," "divine presence," and "god."

Regardless of your religious beliefs or orientation, people who view spirituality (or religion) as important experience greater well-being and lower
risk of unhealthy behaviors, especially among the youth population, than
people who do not. In one large study of over 148,000 middle and high
school students, analysts found that young people who viewed spirituality as important in their lives were 50 percent less likely to use drugs,

40 percent less likely to engage in antisocial behaviors, such as skipping school, and 33 percent less likely to abuse alcohol than peers who did not value spirituality or religion. They were also more likely to exhibit positive behaviors, including higher performance in school and the ability to resist dangerous behaviors, such as driving while under the influence.[3]

As reported in *Handbook of Child Well-Being*, a global study of 6,700 youth aged twelve to twenty-five living across eight countries found that those with an average commitment to spirituality (as defined by nine different measures) fare better than their nonspiritual peers in a number of factors, including happiness, academic success, peaceful conflict resolution, positivity, life satisfaction, and civic and school engagement. What's more, those who value spirituality the most also reported the highest scores across all of these factors.[4]

There are many theories to explain why spiritual and religious people have higher levels of health and happiness. For starters, when these individuals attend regular services at a place of worship, they have a built-in social support network—a factor associated with greater life satisfaction.[5] For youth, these affiliations provide greater opportunities for positive relationships with adults outside their immediate family—a protective factor against risky behaviors and depression. Further, the sense of hope and optimism promoted through spiritual teachings and practices provides individuals with coping skills and support in times of hardship and adversity. Lastly, these individuals also value kindness, community service, and civic engagement—all of which are associated with increased longevity, health, and happiness.

Fortunately, in America, your family is free to practice spirituality and religion in whatever way feels best to you. Bringing any semblance of spirituality to your family life can help children find their sense of purpose, deepen their connections with others, and strengthen their appreciation for all living things.

THE CHANGE
COMMIT TO PRACTICES THAT NURTURE THE SPIRITUAL SELF.

PATH TO CHANGE   Whether or not you are affiliated with an organized religion, getting in touch with and nurturing your personal spirituality can provide many benefits. Consider the following:

DISCOVER YOUR SPIRITUAL TENETS   Start your spiritual journey by identifying what it is you believe and don't believe. One question to start with is "Do you believe in one god, several gods, a higher power, or the philosophy that we are all connected?" Once you answer this question, there are many other factors to consider, such as, "What are the moral principles you would like to embody?" or "Do you believe in heaven, and if so, how would you describe it to your children?" Use the Spiritual Beliefs Worksheet in Part III: Tools and Resources to get started.

WONDER TOGETHER   Parents may shy away from introducing children to spirituality or religion for fear that they may ask questions for which parents don't know the answer. But there is room for uncertainty even in most organized religions. According to a Gallup poll, 75 percent of Americans do not believe that the text in the bible is the actual word of God or that it should be taken literally, but instead believe the bible includes stories inspired by God or are historical examples from which we can learn.[7] Dr. Lisa Miller, author and professor, suggests that when your child asks questions about spiritual or religious concepts for which you have no ready answer, you should resist responding with "I don't know"—an approach that stops the conversation. Instead, try explaining what different people from different religions believe or exploring the topic by asking your child what he thinks.[8]

TEST DRIVE RELIGIOUS OR SPIRITUAL SERVICES   Whether through exposure to friends from different religious backgrounds or natural curiosity, your children may express interest in various religions and practices. It is not uncommon, for instance, for children in middle school to want to attend religious services with their friends' families. Attending services at different houses of worship deepens your child's understanding of the concept of religion and spirituality. Consider attending services with them so you can be part of the exploration process and answer any questions that arise. Most places of worship welcome newcomers and will provide guidance on how to respectfully participate in the service. You can attend services at various churches and temples or learn about other service schedules offered to the public at a local Buddhist temple or ashram.

CREATE SPIRITUAL RITUALS   A 2016 Gallup poll revealed that approximately 48 percent of Americans do not attend religious services regularly, but 75 percent of people feel religion is important to their life. Attending spiritual services that align with your personal beliefs (or family schedule) can be a challenge, but that doesn't preclude your family from embracing practices that nurture spirituality within your home. Consider incorporating the following:

Send love and light Similar to the practice of daily prayer, take a moment each day to send blessings to people you love or individuals who need a little extra support from the universe, a higher power, or god. This practice reinforces that all of us have a responsibility to promote the well-being of others.

Documenting gratitude Regularly writing down a few things for which you are grateful is a practice that promotes happiness, humility, and community. Gratitude is deeply connected to spirituality and can help children reflect on the goodness in their life instead of on things they do not have. Use tips from Week 9, Say Thanks, to explore the practice of gratitude.

Schedule downtime Select a regular day and time for your family to enjoy quiet activities and reflection. For example, use Sunday mornings to write in your journals, do yoga, read a spiritual work, or pray. Do activities with younger children, while letting older children choose activities that meet their own spiritual needs.

Set your intentions At the beginning of many yoga classes, instructors ask participants to set a personal intention for the practice. It is a common request to help yogis experience a deeper connection to their practice and focus their energies toward a defined intention. Similarly, your family can set intentions for each day that help you live out your spiritual goals. Example intentions include: to spread kindness, to be gentle to yourself, to offer understanding to others, or to be strong during difficult times.

Say grace Expressing gratitude before a meal is a simple spiritual act practiced by people from various religions and cultures. Before meals, take a moment to bless the food you will eat. Consider sending thanks to the farmers who grew the food. Thank the earth and sun responsible for providing the soil, nutrients, and energy for growth. And of course, take a moment to express thanks to the individuals who prepared the meal.

PERFORM SERVICE Religious organizations are one of the largest providers of charitable services in the United States. Community service is a spiritual act in that it promotes connection to people in your community, models generosity, and spreads kindness to the world. Find opportunities for your family to donate time to help those in need, using the suggestions from Week 38, Give Back.

GET INTO NATURE   Observing nature and spending time in natural environments reminds us that all living things are connected. Since there are still many unanswered questions associated with the natural world, spending time in these environments can remind us there are many forces bigger than ourselves. See tips from Week 18, Explore Nature, on experiencing nature together.

KNOW YOUR VALUES AND ACTIVELY PRACTICE THEM   Moral values are typically discussed during spiritual or religious services. And children learn about values through stories and activities created by religious teachers and leaders. You can offer similar experiences to your family by engaging in regular discussions about your values and seeking ways to live out values together. Refer to Week 21, Discover Your True North, to learn more about embracing your values.

EMBRACE TRADITION   Simple family traditions can provide a sense of spirituality because they bring together family, friends, and other loved ones around a common belief, activity, or holiday. Create family traditions that provide you and your family with opportunities to explore spirituality. For instance, during Thanksgiving, use the time to express generosity and gratitude as a family by volunteering at a food bank or soup kitchen.

CONQUER ADDED SUGAR

> The longing for sweets is really
> a yearning for love or "sweetness."
> —MARION WOODMAN

WE DON'T NEED science to prove that we love sugar. As infants, our survival depends on an innate desire for sugar, as human milk is extremely sweet. Just one cup of human milk contains almost as much sugar as half a can of regular soda![1] Until the advent of readily available processed sweeteners, once babies were weaned, they adjusted to a diet in which sweets were rare treats. This is no longer the case—and our love affair with sugar is hurting our health. Research connects excess sugar consumption with numerous health conditions, such as increased body weight, hypertension, high cholesterol, diabetes, stroke, cancer, mood disorders, asthma, and gallstones, amongst others.[2,3,4,5] Unfortunately, adults aren't the only ones at risk. Trends indicate a rise in the prevalence of elevated cholesterol, liver inflammation, and type 2 diabetes among children and adolescents in the United States.[6]

Most parents can attest to the noticeable effects sugar has on children's behavior. After a healthy dose of sugary snacks, kids "bounce off the walls" because sugar raises adrenaline. One study found children who eat high-sugar breakfasts have significantly more behavior and attention problems, while another study showed children and adolescents who consumed diets high in refined sugar had lower levels of specific brain proteins, a factor associated with increased risk of depression.[7,8] Beyond mood, sugar also depresses the immune system and creates inflammation, a cause of many diseases and conditions.

Every cell in your body uses glucose (sugar) for energy. In order for the sugar to enter those cells, insulin levels increase when sugar is ingested. When we chronically consume more sugar than we need, however, excess insulin is converted to triglycerides and stored as fat, usually in the abdomen. And because insulin promotes the storage of fat, it can become a vicious cycle. Eventually, cells no longer respond to insulin, leading to insulin resistance and chronically high blood sugar. Though families may not be overeating table sugar by the spoonful, research shows we are chronically consuming an excess of added sugar, usually hidden in processed foods.[9]

DID YOU KNOW?

The American Heart Association (AHA) recommends that children ages two to eighteen should consume no more than 6 teaspoons, or 25 grams, of added sugar daily, and no more than 8 ounces of sugar-sweetened beverages weekly. Similarly, AHA recommends women consume no more than 6 teaspoons daily, and men no more than 9 teaspoons.[10]

Modifying sugar intake as a family will have long-term benefits because eating behaviors acquired in childhood persist into adulthood.[11] Further, research shows that parents have great influence over the eating patterns and preferences of children, even adolescents. Studies show children of authoritative parents—a parenting style recognized for setting limits and clear expectations—eat more fruit per day and fewer unhealthy snacks, and they eat breakfast more often than children of other parenting styles.[12,13] By reducing sugar intake, both parents and children lower their risk of preventable health conditions.

THE CHANGE
REDUCE ADDED SUGAR INTAKE.

PATH TO CHANGE   Reducing sugar intake is one of the most important steps your family can take to achieve a healthy lifestyle. This will take time, but the following tips should ease the process:

BY THE NUMBERS   The nutrition facts label, found on packaged foods and beverages, provides a summary of the nutrient content contained in a product. "Sugars" appears under "Total Carbohydrate" and refers to the quantity of sugar (in grams) found in one serving of the food. In this example, the entire package makes up one serving and contains 23 grams of sugars.

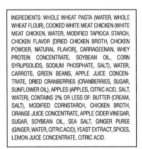

Nutrition Label and Ingredients List[14]

BUY THE INGREDIENTS   Below the nutrition facts label you will find the ingredient list, containing all ingredients found in a product, including sweeteners. Manufacturers use over sixty different names for sweeteners, so it can get confusing. Aim to have as few sweeteners as possible (or ideally, none) in any packaged product you consume.

BE SUGAR DETECTIVES   A study by the Centers for Disease Control found that 90 percent of added sugar intake consumed by Americans comes from ultra-processed foods, such as soft drinks, fruit drinks, baked goods, breakfast cereals, snacks, and ice cream.[15] Since sugar lurks in packaged foods, it's best to evaluate the sugar content in your family's favorites. Engage the family in finding sugar together by evaluating every packaged product, including products you may not think contain added sugar, such as tomato sauce, soup, bread, taco shells, crackers, nut butter, milk, milk alternatives, and dressing.

CONQUER SUGAR CRAVINGS   Once administered only by pharmacists in the 1500s in Europe, sugar is found to be more addictive to the brain than cocaine and other drugs.[16,17] Instead of turning to harmful alternatives such as artificial sweeteners, which are proven to increase both weight and cravings and cause cancer, help your family reduce sugar cravings naturally. Serve balanced meals, consume adequate amounts of healthy fat, get high-quality sleep, and reduce actual sugar intake.[18] If you or a family member has an addiction to sugar or artificial sweeteners, consider working with a functional nutritionist to identify and address the root cause of the cravings.

Juice and juice cocktails   Most fruit juice mixes include other sweeteners and fillers, but even those labeled as 100 percent juice typically contain just as much sugar as a soda. Opt for green juice that is slightly sweetened with low-sugar fruits including apples and berries.

Sports drinks   Most drinks marketed to athletes are loaded with artificial sweeteners and/or added sugar. Also, many "healthy" flavored water-based drinks contain high sugar content or artificial sweeteners.

Coffee drinks   Fancy coffee drinks prepared by your favorite barista can contain up to 60 grams of sugar! Skip the syrups and add-ins to avoid artificial sweeteners and excess sugar.

Flavored tea   Powdered and bottled teas can contain a lot of sugar. One 16-ounce bottle typically contains two servings, so double the grams of sugar listed if you drink the entire bottle.

HIDDEN CULPRITS   Packaged foods containing more than five ingredients often include multiple forms of sugar and/or artificial sweeteners. As we wrote this book, we found over sixty different names for sugar, with manufacturers creating new ones regularly. Since sugar can have many aliases, avoid products containing more than five to ten ingredients.

Flavored yogurt   Most fruit-based yogurts contain added sugar in addition to fruit and yogurt. Some of the most popular brands contain upwards of 25 grams of sugar!

Condiments   On average, Americans consume 3 tablespoons of ketchup with each burger and fries. This equates to a whopping 12 to 15 grams of sugar! Condiments, such as ketchup and barbecue sauce, and premade salad dressings are typically high in sugar.

Cereal   Packaged cereal is one of the most sugary products on the market. Further, healthy marketing claims, such as "good source of fiber" or "helps lower cholesterol" mask high levels of unhealthy added sugar. A large study conducted by the Environmental Working Group evaluated the sugar content in over 1,500 cereals, including 181 marketed to children. EWG researchers found that 34 percent of calories in children's cereals are from added sugars. Also, in 40 of the 181 cereals marketed to children, a single serving contained over 60 percent of the daily limit of sugar recommended by health organizations.[19]

Granola and protein bars Often marketed as a healthy, portion-controlled option, protein bars and granola bars contain high amounts of sugar. Though some versions are sweetened with dried fruit, a healthier alternative, many contain sweeteners in syrup form to keep the bars from falling apart.

SEEK HEALTHIER ALTERNATIVES   Depending on your children's ages, if you suddenly stop buying their favorite foods you may get a lot of pushback. Help children find healthier alternatives by visiting the grocery store together and reading nutrition labels of similar products. Although many products found in the natural/organic sections of the grocery store are healthier, it's important to read the labels to be sure. The best way to choose healthy products is to choose alternatives that are whole food–based. For example, choose apples or unsweetened applesauce in place of sweetened applesauce. Refer to the Healthy Food Swaps table later in this chapter for some ideas.

COOK AND BAKE AT HOME   Families who cook and bake at home have much more control over the sugar content in their food. When you cook, adjust recipes calling for sugary condiments by adding just a little at a time until you reach a desired level of sweetness. To find healthier versions of your favorite baking recipes, use search terms such as paleo (typically no grains, legumes, or refined sugar), low added sugar, healthy, and/or grain-free.

UNDERSTAND MODERATION   Restricting all sugary foods will create a feeling of deprivation, only increasing cravings for these foods. Follow the preceding suggestions to find healthier alternatives for the most prominent high-sugar foods in your family's diet. And for those absolute favorites, choose specific times to enjoy them. For example, families may choose to go out for ice cream once per week rather than enjoying ice cream treats daily.

HEALTHY FOOD SWAPS

SUGARY FOOD	HEALTHIER ALTERNATIVE
Cereal	Unsweetened hot cereal, such as oatmeal, topped with fruit Homemade muesli (whole rolled oats, nuts, seeds, dried fruit, coconut flakes)
Coffee drinks	Homemade "bulletproof" coffee (coffee, unsweetened almond milk, grass-fed butter or coconut oil, vanilla extract)
Cookies	Homemade cookie bites (combine 1 cup [1g]oats, 2 bananas, and ¼ cup [45g] chocolate chips, mix well, and drop teaspoons of dough onto parchment-lined baking sheet; bake at 350°F [175°C] for 10 to 15 minutes.) Trail mix with chocolate chips
Fruit-flavored yogurt	Unsweetened, full-fat yogurt with fresh fruit on top (even a little honey goes a long way)
Fruit juice	Whole fruit Water infused with crushed fruit Herbal fruit-based tea
Fruit snacks	Dehydrated fruit Unsweetened dried fruit, such as cherries or apples
Drinkable yogurt	Kefir pureed with fruit and a bit of honey or maple syrup
Graham crackers	Pumpkin seeds dusted with cinnamon and date sugar Brown rice cake spread with nut butter and dusted with cinnamon
Granola bars	Trail mix with nuts, seeds, and some dried fruit Homemade muesli (see Cereal)
Soda	Flavored seltzer Seltzer and fruit-flavored tea

LOVE TO DO, NOT TO HAVE

Happiness resides not in possessions, and not
in gold; happiness dwells in the soul.
—DEMOCRITUS

WHETHER IT'S APPLE products or *Star Wars* gear, adults and children alike
can be seduced by the never-ending cycle of consumerism that clutters
our homes and our lives. But is all this stuff bringing us happiness?

According to psychologists and researchers, we experience more enjoyment and positive emotion from the purchase of an experience than
from the purchase of a material possession.[1] As time passes, enthusiasm
for these possessions wanes, while our emotional connection to experiential purchases grows. So often, children beg for a new toy or gadget,
only to get it and start begging for another within weeks or even days.
With time, new things lose their novelty and become part of everyday
life, providing us with only a short-lived feeling of joy or satisfaction.
Even when we take moments to appreciate all that we have, it's natural
to take our material "stuff" for granted.

Experiences, on the other hand, establish memories that can be invoked
repeatedly over time, bringing unlimited joy. With time we actually

remember our experiences more favorably than what we originally felt—we tend to forget the mishaps and focus on the positive. And since experiences are often shared with others rather than alone, they bring us even more joy. Another reason experiences bring more joy and happiness is because they are often shared with others rather than alone.[2] The sharing of experiences enhances our relationships and forges new bonds with people—both of which contribute to our happiness.

_____

DID YOU KNOW?

Only 3.1 percent of the world's children live in America, but America's children own 40 percent of all the toys produced globally.[3]

_____

Pursuing happiness through material possessions leads to a never-ending cycle and a void that seems to never be filled. As parents, we have the power to model and teach children how to embrace all that life has to offer by seeking experiences that create a lifetime of memories.

THE CHANGE
PURSUE EXPERIENCES OVER POSSESSIONS.

PATH TO CHANGE   Families who seek experiences over possessions can cut down on clutter in their homes and open the door to new opportunities. Use the following strategies to help your family shift to valuing experiences over possessions:

BECOME MINDFUL OF PURCHASES   Every time a family member requests a new possession that is not a necessity, discuss the reasons behind the desire and evaluate the cost and benefits together. Parents can model this approach by consciously sharing their own process for making purchasing decisions.

Get to the root need Take time to understand what the possession will fulfill for yourself or your child. Abraham Maslow's famous hierarchy of needs theory says that human beings have five needs: physiological, safety, love/belonging, self-esteem, and self-actualization—each need must be met before humans desire the next need in the hierarchy.[4] Which need does the possession fill for you or you child? Understand the importance of the possession and determine if there are other factors at play that need to be addressed. For example, if a teen wants the latest tech gadget, it may be because she wants to feel cool or accepted by a specific group of kids. In this instance, helping your teen strengthen her sense of belonging by spending more time with friends, new and old, will bring her more sustained joy than purchasing a new gadget that loses its luster within days.

Experience-based alternatives We can all appreciate the old adage "Money doesn't grow on trees," but do we really follow its intent? Your family can increase appreciation for the cost of goods when you start considering the alternatives. When a new possession is requested, discuss the ways in which the same amount of money can be used toward purchases that are more experiential and have longer-lasting benefits instead. For example, your child may prefer to attend a sporting event instead of getting the newest athletic jersey.

Learn about manufacturing Another way to help your family understand and appreciate the value of their things is to learn how different objects are made. You can watch documentaries such as *True Cost* about the fast fashion industry, or *The Story of Stuff* about how we make and throw away things, or find YouTube videos on this topic.

Find a nearby flea market Flea markets are filled with mounds of unwanted, useless stuff people are trying to sell before they give up and dump it. Use this trip as as an opportunity to show how one person's trash can become another person's treasure!

REDUCE THE VALUE YOU PLACE ON OWNERSHIP OF THINGS If your family is used to owning the latest and greatest toys, gadgets, and books, you can wean yourselves off this mentality by focusing on reusing items instead of purchasing new. Make it a game and a family event to find ways to borrow or buy used goods.

Borrow from the library Public libraries are starting to offer patrons the opportunity to borrow more than just books. Many libraries have toys, games, and even cookware that you can borrow.

Swap with friends Most women can remember sharing clothes with friends when they were teenagers. Try promoting this approach for clothing and other items, such as books, movies, kitchen gadgets, and toys. Start by sharing your family's plan to reduce purchases with a small group of friends or neighbors, and see if anyone is willing to try a swap. The best part of a swap is that you become much closer with those willing to participate.

One in, one out Try creating a family rule that requires everyone to donate something each time a new material possession is purchased. You can exclude collectibles such as books, movies, and music.

START FAMILY BUCKET LISTS   Create a bucket list containing all of the experiences your family would like to enjoy together. Allow all family members to add to the bucket list, and keep it visible so everyone is inspired to save money and plan for new experiences. Make your bucket list a reality by creating a "family experience" jar or a jar dedicated to saving up the funds for your family's next adventure. Each week, talk with your family about the money you each chose to divert from other purchases, so they can be inspired to save money as well.

COMMEMORATE EXPERIENCES   Reminiscing about experiences brings continuous joy and keeps these memories alive in our minds. Don't let an experience go undocumented. Try the following ideas to memorialize them:

Share photos With smartphones, it is highly likely a camera is always within arm's reach. Take photos to remember experiences, and share them with friends and family via text or social media.

Print photo books Most photo printing companies, such as Shutterfly and even CVS, offer apps that make printing photos or photo books a breeze. You can upload photos to one of these websites or via a smartphone app to create a photo book that documents the entire experience.

Create a family journal Flipping through pages of photo albums or journals is one of the most tangible ways to bring past experiences alive. Use a sturdy notebook or scrapbook to document your family's memories, or purchase a photo album that you can write in to make it more robust. Make it an annual affair to update the journal together!

SHARE THE FUN   Enjoy experiences with friends, family, and neighbors. Your family will deepen their relationships with those involved through the extra time spent together, while creating a new memory to reminisce about during future gatherings.

USE EXPERIENCES TO CELEBRATE   Typically, families celebrate birthdays, holidays, and graduations with tangible gifts, but using experiences can be even more fulfilling. Plan an experience together in addition to a small gift (or in lieu of any gifts, if all family members agree) for a typical gift-giving occasion. For instance, if your child is graduating from high school, forgo a graduation gift, and instead throw a big party or plan a trip as a family to a destination of their choice. Children will continue to remember the experiences for years to come.

SURF AND SOCIALIZE ONLINE SAFELY

The Internet is becoming the town square
for the global village of tomorrow.

—BILL GATES

OUR CHILDREN LIVE in a very different technological world than the one we grew up in. Dubbed "Generation I" by Bill Gates and "Re-generation" by award-winning author Tammy Erickson, today's children are the first generation to have access to everything, everywhere, at every time of the day, due to the proliferation of wireless technology, mobile devices, and unlimited content.[1]

In fact, a 2013 research study by Common Sense Media found that 72 percent of children under age eight and 38 percent of children under age two have used a mobile device for watching videos, playing games, or using apps.[2] Another study, by the Pew Research Center, found 24 percent of teens report being "online constantly" and 56 percent go online several times per day. These statistics are not surprising, given that 73 percent of teens and 77 percent of adults have access to smartphones.[3,4] And with most adults relying on connectivity for work, access to family and friends, and household management, it's almost certain we'd be lost without mobile devices and wireless internet access.

With the all-pervasive Internet, it's imperative we protect our children from the many hidden dangers of the online world. Almost one in five adolescents experience cyber bullying, online contact with strangers, sexual messaging, or unwanted exposure to pornography.[5] Various studies also find between 25 and 42 percent of children encounter unwanted sexually explicit content when searching online.[6] One study by the Kaiser Family Foundation found 70 percent of children ages eight to eighteen were exposed to sexual content when searching online for health information.[7] According to a review of several studies, chronic exposure to pornography and sexually explicit material (regardless of age) contributes to a multitude of negative effects, from more sexually permissive attitudes to less satisfaction with one's own sexual life.[8]

Identity theft is another concern, hitting an all-time high in 2016 when $16 billion was stolen from more than fifteen million U.S. consumers.[9] According to Carnegie Mellon CyLab report, researchers found the identity theft rate of children to be fifty-one times that of adults during the same time period.[10] It's not uncommon for apps and gaming websites to request personal information, making younger children, who are uneducated about the dangers of sharing personal information online, more susceptible.

Fortunately, many schools are incorporating internet safety education into traditional curricula. The content accessed at schools and libraries is often highly filtered (per the Children's Internet Protection Act). Therefore a typical web search would not result in sexually explicit content that might appear on an unfiltered home computer. Other websites commonly containing explicit content (such as YouTube) are also not accessible at schools or libraries. This protects children in these settings, but that safety may give both children and their parents a false sense of security. Thus parents need to take additional steps to teach their families about internet safety at home.

Learning and teaching children about internet safety can reduce risk of harm, create an open dialogue about online activity, and give your children confidence about using the Internet. A recent study from EU Kids found that when parents "actively mediate" the Internet use of children, the risk of online victimization declines considerably. Active mediation includes talking with children about the Internet, staying nearby or sitting with them while they go online, encouraging them to explore the Internet, and sharing online activities with them.[11] Active mediation is preferred to restriction because children are still afforded opportunities to gain knowledge and important digital skills needed in the twenty-first century.

DID YOU KNOW?

The legal consequences of "sexting" are often not fully understood by children or their parents. Possession of a sexually explicit image of a minor is a crime. Sending that image to another minor is also a crime. And coercing or soliciting someone to send a sexually explicit image is a crime. In states that do not have specific sexting laws, officials will rely on tough child pornography laws to determine avenues of prosecution, including jail time.[12]

THE CHANGE
EDUCATE YOUR FAMILY ON INTERNET SAFETY AND ACTIVELY MEDIATE INTERNET ACTIVITY OF YOUNGER CHILDREN.

PATH TO CHANGE   Use the following steps to increase online safety in your household and protect your family from victimization:

ACTIVELY MEDIATE YOUNGER CHILDREN   Research finds that children are safer online when parents are more engaged with their behaviors and activity. Sit with or nearby children when they are using smartphones or the Internet. Use the opportunity to teach them how to avoid in-app purchases and inappropriate content and how to stay safe. They'll be appreciative when you help them find content that aligns with their interests and expands their skills.

BE PARTNERS When children become savvy about using the computer and the Internet for schoolwork and social communication, it may seem our parental role is no longer necessary, but many would argue our continued presence is even more important. Establish a partnership with your children that gives them independence, but also your ongoing support. For example, join the same social networking sites and become friends online. Engage in their posts, share interesting content that aligns with their interests, and get to know their friends—take the same parental role online as you do in everyday life. Explain to children that being partners means helping one another out—whether he teaches you how to use a new app or you provide her with advice about a sticky situation.

SET SAFE PARAMETERS Maintaining safety on the Internet becomes much more difficult as children get older and spend more time away from you. Work together to set age-appropriate parameters that keep your family safe. For example, set all devices to forget the Wi-Fi password so children need to check in before they go online.

Common areas According to Media Smarts, over 60 percent of teens have posed as an adult online to register for adult-specific websites. Require that all online activities occur in common areas so you can be available to guide children through any issues that arise, such as avoiding uncomfortable content or handling requests for personal information.

Making online friends Shockingly, 57 percent of teens make new friends online.[13] Accepting friend requests from people you do not know gives strangers access to information such as where you live or hang out, or when you're away on vacation. This increases your family's risk of identity theft and even burglary. Regularly review your children's personal list of friends on social media platforms so you can work together to keep their content private.

ONLINE AT EVERY AGE[14]

AGE	SAFETY PRECAUTIONS	DISCUSSION TOPICS
5 to 7 years	Block pop-ups. Use ad-blocking software. Choose kid-friendly search engines. Bookmark age-appropriate sites. Set a password for all purchases. Go online with children or sit next to them when online.	Not providing any personal information online Communicating when you find scary or confusing content
8 to 10 years	Require online activities be performed in common family areas. Use family email accounts. Preview content and websites first. Understand parental controls of all devices that go on the Internet. Practice social networking using a family social networking page. Provide basic cell phone without internet access. Start a regular dialogue about uncomfortable or questionable content.	Safe and ethical social networking (not sharing passwords, uploading photos with permission) Online posts and pictures Requests for personal information Online friends vs. real friends
11 to 13 years	Designate tech-free zones in the bedroom and at the dining table. Online activity in common areas. Teach "safe" search features. Consider allowing personal social networking pages. Join chat rooms or websites your children use. Become friends online.	Cyberbullying Online predators Privacy settings Online footprint Pornography Safe sites for music Online friends Identify theft/personal information
14 to 17 years	Continue tech-free zones. Keep online activities in common areas. Continue as friends with children online.	Right to privacy Cyberbullying Sexting laws Illegal downloading Predators Identity theft/online financial purchases

Keep personal information private Online thieves can access your financial institution and personal records by tracking any personal information entered online. Even an email address doubled as a user ID can be used to gain access to your identity. Talk with your family about these risks and set rules for consulting with an adult when sharing personal information online, including email addresses.

CONSIDER MONITORING SOFTWARE   Monitoring a child's online activity tends to be a controversial topic. Some parents feel that monitoring invades a child's privacy; others believe monitoring is a must, given the vast array of hidden dangers in cyberspace. The monitoring programs and apps available now range from more comprehensive versions that cover all aspects of online activity to highly specific versions that focus on one particular area of activity, such as tracking cell use. Instead of spying on children, use your findings as an opportunity to have conversations about online activity.

DELAY SMARTPHONE OWNERSHIP   When surveyed, many technology leaders claim their children do not receive personal smartphones until eighth grade or fourteen years old. A group of concerned parents created an initiative (www.Waituntil8th.org) encouraging parents to join together and pledge they will wait until eighth grade to provide a child with a smartphone. To learn more about the detrimental effects of excess screen time, read Week 8, Make Screen Time Purposeful.

LOVE YOUR BODY

People often say that "beauty is in the eye of the beholder," and I say that the most liberating thing about beauty is realizing that you are the beholder.

—SALMA HAYEK

IT IS VIRTUALLY impossible to ignore the gaping differences between the bodies of real people and the airbrushed images of perfection featured on television, billboards, product packaging, and toys. These unrealistic images of beauty and body shape can take a tremendous toll on our own body image and self-esteem. Unfortunately, body dissatisfaction can begin as early as childhood and persist throughout life. One study by Common Sense Media found that children as young as five years old expressed discontent with their bodies.[1]

According to the National Eating Disorders Association (NEDA), girls as young as six years old become aware of their own body shape and begin articulating concerns about it. By the time they reach elementary school, 40 to 60 percent of girls are worried about becoming too fat or gaining weight.[2] At this age, however, girls should be focused on having fun, playing, learning, and loving life, rather than stressing about their body shape.

Although not as commonly discussed, boys' body image is similarly affected by the unattainable image of perfection. Not only do airbrushed images of females subconsciously shape boys' definition of beauty, but the large, lean, and muscular body shapes that dominate action figures and superheroes distort boys' views of masculinity. In one study of almost 1,300 adolescent boys (grades six to twelve), 35 percent of boys admitted to using protein powders or shakes, 6 percent used steroids, and 10 percent used other muscle-enhancing substances to increase muscle mass and tone.[6] These behaviors are especially disturbing, as we know that adolescent boys with muscularity and weight anxieties are more likely to develop highly depressive symptoms, use drugs, and binge drink.[7]

Fortunately, parents aren't powerless in the fight to raise body-positive children. Though we can't change the images featured in movies, magazines, books, and toys, we can shift our own attitudes, language, purchasing habits, and topics of conversation to create a more body-positive environment for our children. Research indicates it's even more imperative that we improve our own body image in order to help our children feel content and confident with their personal body. For example, studies show time and time again that a mother's level of dissatisfaction with her body image is directly correlated to her child's level of dissatisfaction with her own body image. Other studies show that fathers who provide encouragement and nurturance to their children and avoid body shape jokes can instill self-confidence in boys and girls, protecting them from body image concerns.

THE CHANGE
CREATE A POSITIVE BODY IMAGE ENVIRONMENT.

PATH TO CHANGE   Creating an environment that encourages your family members to love their bodies and avoid comparing themselves to the unrealistic images of Hollywood and other media will be crucial in helping your children develop healthy body awareness. Use the following effective strategies:

HEALTHY ROLE MODELS   Every prominent adult in your child's life, from the voice coach to the swim coach, can affect your child's body image. Find role models that promote a love of self, and focus on skill, talent, and attitudes rather than appearance. Be wary of teams or activities that require children to weigh in, track food intake, or take specific supplements. If your child participates in activities that require a certain physique or weight, such as wrestling, seek professional help from a psychologist or social worker to understand how these requirements can affect your child.

PRACTICE SELF CARE   There are many ways we care for and protect our bodies. And doing so lays down a strong foundation for self-love and positive self-esteem. Wearing a helmet while riding a bike or a seat belt in the car, brushing our teeth, staying hydrated, eating healthy food, staying active, and getting plenty of rest are all simple ways we can take good care of our bodies and promote healthy self-esteem.

BANISH CRITICAL BODY TALK   Children soak up everything we do and say, even the negative self-talk we mumble under our breath when we don't like how we look in the mirror. Talking negatively about your own appearance or the appearance of others can cause your children to be more conscious and hypercritical of their appearance. Be sure to make comments about yourself and others either neutral or positive. This not only benefits your children but also helps keep you in a more self-loving mindset.

USE ANATOMICALLY CORRECT LANGUAGE It can seem cute or funny, or feel easier or more comfortable to call your child's genitals "winkie" or "hoohoo" instead of penis and vagina, but it creates confusion for children. Using the correct terms for genitals helps children understand their bodies so they can ask questions about their development. It also reinforces the need to respect your private body parts and those of others, rather than allowing them to be the source of laughter. Lastly, when young children use correct vocabulary for genitals, they can protect themselves from abuse and report inappropriate touching using terms that are understood by other adults.

TALK ABOUT BODY CHANGES Preparing children for body changes that will occur before, during, and after puberty will empower them and instill confidence in understanding and anticipating their own development. The changes associated with the onset of puberty can start as early as age eight, so you should discuss with them at around this age. You can make your child more comfortable by using age-appropriate books on anatomy and physiology in your discussions. And fictional books, such as *Are You There, God? It's Me, Margaret*, for girls, or, for boys, *Then Again, Maybe I Won't* are great examples of stories that cover sensitive topics, such as breast development and menstruation, in a fun-loving way.

GO BEYOND THE SURFACE It's normal for young children to notice how people look by observing opposites such as "tall" and "short." Instead of focusing on appearances, however, discuss nonphysical traits of individuals. Talk about the strength and speed of famous athletes or the precision of a musician. Explain how they achieved their success through long hours of dedicated effort and hard work. Discuss with tweens and teens that it's more important to be strong and fit than to be thin. And instead of focusing on appearances of favorite pop stars, explain the exercise regimen and hard work they go through to achieve their look.

TEACH RESPECT   Schools set rules and spend a lot of time teaching children to respect their bodies and the bodies of others. Preschoolers learn to ask permission before hugging or kissing another child, while teens learn the concept of consensual sex. Extending these lessons within your home reinforces that your family supports these values as well. Teach siblings to check in with each other before wrestling, and allow children to make their own decisions regarding showing affection to family members, such as kissing their grandmother and grandfather.

SEEK A PROFESSIONAL   A national survey of over ten thousand adolescents found 6.1 percent of boys and girls suffer from clinical eating disorders or symptoms that may indicate an eating issue.[8] Eating disorders are complex conditions that often start with preoccupations with food and weight. If any family member has overtly negative feelings about her body, constantly compares herself to others, severely restricts food, or experiences unshakable negative feelings from the weight she sees on the scale, it may be beneficial to seek therapy from a psychologist or social worker who specializes in body image.

GO FISH

Fish in the hands of a skilled cook can become an
inexhaustible source of gustatory pleasures.
—JEAN-ANTHELEME BRILLAT-SAVARIN

FISH IS A high-quality protein that is low in saturated fat and contains
important micronutrients, such as vitamins B12 and D, selenium, potassium, magnesium, and calcium. Most important, fish and seafood are
high in omega-3 fats.

Omega-3 fats improve heart health by reducing the risk of blood clots,
decreasing triglyceride levels, slowing the growth of plaques in the blood
vessels, making arteries more flexible, and lowering inflammation. They
also benefit brain health for similar reasons—they improve blood flow,
lower inflammation, and reduce the aggregation of proteins, a major
cause of Alzheimer's disease. Their role in brain function is especially
helpful for lowering risk of dementia, depression, and cognitive decline,
and improving focus and memory.[1,2]

Since these essential fatty acids are not produced in the body, we must get
them through our diet. Many plant foods, such as walnuts and flaxseed,
contain omega-3s called ALA (alpha-linolenic acid). To see the positive
health benefits from omega-3s, however, the body must convert ALA
into long chain fatty acids, called DHA (docosahexaenoic acid) and EPA

(eicosapentaenoic acid). But this process is inefficient and does not provide the body with adequate levels of DHA and EPA. Fortunately, fish contains both DHA and EPA. Americans, however, are falling short on intake of fish. Per recent estimates, the average American eats only 4.77 ounces weekly, which is far from the 8 to 12 ounces weekly recommended by the USDA.[3]

Put simply, omega-3 fats found in fish and seafood are critical to your family's health and well-being. (Vegetarians and vegans who don't eat fish are advised to take a high-quality supplement.)

THE CHANGE
AIM TO EAT FISH AND SEAFOOD LOW IN MERCURY THREE TIMES PER WEEK.

PATH TO CHANGE   Use the following tips to incorporate healthier fish into your family's diet:

UNDERSTAND METHYL MERCURY   Mercury is a naturally occurring chemical found in deposits of coal and released into the air through industrial pollution. Because it accumulates in oceans and streams where fish live, nearly all fish and seafood contain traces of mercury. The larger, longer-lived predatory fish have the highest levels because of their prolonged exposure. Mercury in all its forms is toxic to humans, especially to a developing fetus. For example, one study found that pregnant women with the highest blood mercury levels gave birth to children with the lowest development scores measured at age three.[4] People who consume too much fish that is high in mercury can experience damage to the central nervous system. This can result in difficulty with memory and concentration, headaches, fatigue, and more. Choose more low-mercury seafood varieties, especially when pregnant.[5]

FARMED FISH   Research has found that farmed fish is more fatty and therefore has much higher concentrations of several toxic pollutants, including polychlorinated biphenyls (PCBs), pesticides, and carcinogenic chemicals, all of which accumulate in the fat of the fish.[6] Not all fish farming practices around the world operate the same way. Whole Foods Market sources responsibly farmed seafood. Check their website for a complete listing of their standards so you can feel comfortable with the health profile of these farmed fish options (www.wholefoodsmarket.com /farm-raised-seafood).

GO WILD   Since wild fish aren't kept in constricted environments, they are not treated with pesticides or antibiotics. Choose wild seafood to reduce exposure to these harmful chemicals. The Monterey Bay Aquarium has a Seafood Watch program and app that provides up-to-date science-based sustainability ratings for all fish species.

ENJOY FATTY FISH   Wild fatty fish—such as wild salmon, sardines, anchovies, and herring—provide significantly higher levels of the heart-healthy, brain-boosting omega-3 essential fatty acids with lower levels of mercury.

SAFE WITH SUSHI   Typically, prepared sushi purchased in grocery stores and most restaurants contains farmed fish and is likely not a sustainable choice. Choose vegetarian options whenever possible, or make sushi a rare treat for your family. If you have a local favorite sushi restaurant, talk with the chef about your interest in low-mercury, sustainably caught varieties.

CHOOSE SAFE SEAFOOD

THIS TABLE PRESENTS a simple, short list of common seafood varieties categorized according to levels of toxic mercury and healthy omega-3 fats.[7]

BEST CHOICES	GOOD CHOICES	SAFE CHOICES	CONCERNING CHOICES	UNSAFE CHOICES
Sustainable Low mercury Highest omega-3s	Low mercury High omega-3s	Low mercury Good omega-3s	High mercury	Very high mercury Must be avoided by pregnant women and children
Wild salmon Sardines Mussels Rainbow trout Atlantic mackerel	Oysters Anchovies Pollock Herring	Shrimp Catfish Tilapia Clams Scallops	Canned tuna Halibut Lobster Mahi mahi Sea bass	Shark Swordfish Tilefish King mackerel Marlin Bluefin tuna Bigeye tuna Orange roughy

Source: Environmental Working Group

RESPECT DIFFERENCES

> An individual has not started living until he can
> rise above the narrow confines of his individualistic
> concerns to the broader concerns of all humanity.
> —MARTIN LUTHER KING, JR.

INTERNATIONAL MIGRATION HAS grown rapidly since the turn of the twenty-first century. Over 244 million people have migrated from their country of birth to another area of the world, with the majority of migrants living in high-income countries such as the United States and Canada, the United Kingdom, and the United Arab Emirates. Cultural diversity is one of the many benefits that international migrants provide their host countries.[1] As the largest host of international migrants world-wide, the United States is more racially and ethnically diverse than ever before, and according to projections, it will become even more so in the next half century.[2]

Beyond diversity of race and ethnicity, gender diversity is on the rise as well. In 2016, 4.1 percent of Americans identified as lesbian, gay, bisexual, or transgender—a 21 percent increase in just four years.[3]

Our increasingly diverse world requires people to be more tolerant and open-minded. Fortunately, these traits are also associated with better health and success. People who are more open-minded, especially in learning environments, are more flexible thinkers—a coveted characteristic in the constantly changing technology industry.[4] Tolerant individuals are also more successful in dealing with life changes. In fact, longitudinal studies find people with psychological flexibility or open-mindedness have better mental health and a lower probability of psychiatric issues.[5] Researchers theorize that individuals with psychological flexibility enjoy better health for a variety of reasons. For starters, they are better able to modify their behaviors in constantly changing situations. They can also endure more pain and recover more rapidly from pain-inducing situations. And flexible individuals have a stronger ability to shift how they spend their time to maintain better well-being.[6] Overall, people who are open-minded exhibit greater well-being and have healthier outcomes in life.[7,8]

Corporate environments that embrace diversity also benefit. In one study, researchers found innovative financial institutions with the most racially diverse workforce had much higher financial performance than organizations with less diversity.[9] Further, decades of research show that groups of people with diverse backgrounds are more creative and innovative in their work.[10]

It is possible to increase your tolerance and open-mindedness, regardless of your age. And parents who take conscious steps to raise open-minded children will provide them with tools for being more successful at every life stage and wherever they live in the world.

DID YOU KNOW?

Individuals who are highly open to new ideas, experiences, and interests can detect stimuli in their environment that other people cannot. Researchers find open-minded people are less likely to experience "inattentional blindness"—a phenomenon in which people do not see unexpected objects that appear because their attention is focused elsewhere.[11] This research shows that our personality traits can also impact our visual perception.

THE CHANGE
TEACH OPEN-MINDEDEDNESS AND APPRECIATION FOR DIVERSITY OF RACE, ETHNICITY, RELIGION, SEXUAL ORIENTATION, AND GENDER IDENTITY.

PATH TO CHANGE   Use the following strategies to help your family adopt an open mind and appreciate diversity:

TALK ABOUT DIVERSITY   Research shows that children as young as three months can recognize diversity in people. Infants tend to stare longer at people who look racially and ethnically similar to their family and caregivers.[12] Christopher Metzler, an expert in diversity and inclusion, tells families it is imperative to talk about diversity-related topics in order to help children understand and appreciate the differences they notice about other people.[13] When we don't talk about diversity, naturally curious children will be left with unanswered questions and may be more easily influenced by intolerant viewpoints.

HAVE A DIVERSE INNER CIRCLE   By spending time with people who come from backgrounds different than your own, your family will not only learn about a variety of lifestyles and traditions but also become more familiar and comfortable with diversity. Depending on where you live, connecting with people from different races or religions may require more effort. Attend religious services at a racially diverse church or one that welcomes the lesbian, gay, bisexual, and transgender (LGBT) population. Or introduce yourself to, and connect with, diverse professionals you often see at the grocery store, the post office, or your regular gas station.

ATTEND MULTICULTURAL EVENTS   Festivals and events created to celebrate a specific racial or ethnic group are fun, entertaining, and educational. Most events feature traditional food, music, dances, and history of the people being celebrated. For example, go to events celebrating Black

History Month (February), Chinese New Year (February), Asian Pacific American History Month (May), or National American Indian Heritage Month (November).

REVISIT HISTORY   Using a historical lens to explore diversity provides an educational component. Explore your library for age-appropriate stories that are historically accurate. Visit museums to teach children about the language, history, and lifestyle of people from various cultures, religions, and countries. Although race and religious persecution are highly sensitive topics, discussing them openly and honestly with children allows them to develop empathy and a deeper understanding of how to respect and appreciate diversity. Ask your librarian for inclusive book recommendations.

PRACTICE RESPECTFUL DISAGREEMENT   People from varying backgrounds naturally bring different perspectives and ideas to the table. Understanding how to listen to others and respectfully disagree with their viewpoints is a highly valuable skill. You can model this by having mock arguments with children or demonstrating these concepts during play with younger children. Psychologist and author Dr. Erica Reischer explains that parents can teach children how to share their opinions while considering someone else's opinion without making the other person feel devalued or disrespected.[14]

TEMPER LANGUAGE   It's easy to express frustration about supporters of the opposing political party or feel negatively toward fans of a rival sports team. Though we may not realize it, our children become highly attuned to the language, word choice, and tone we use when referencing people who think differently from us. Young children are especially vulnerable to these situations because they cannot always discern the difference between joking and cruel heckling. Help children understand how to be respectful fans and supporters without resorting to rude language or unkind insults.

GO BEYOND
THE PIGGY BANK

The art is not in making money, but in keeping it.
—PROVERB

FINANCIAL RESPONSIBILITY MAY not be a traditional habit to practice for good health, but it's one of extreme importance. Like other stressors, concerns and worry over money have a direct impact on your family's health. For example, studies have found that people who report financial problems of indebtedness and financial stress also report symptoms of depression, anxiety, and anger.[1,2] And age is irrelevant. According to a study of 8,400 young adults aged twenty-four to thirty-two, household debt was found to be a significant predictor of poorer health outcomes. The study showed that even in this young age group, higher debt was significantly associated with increased blood pressure and prevalence of symptoms of depression.

There is a huge debt crisis in America right now. In May 2017, U.S. consumers owed $764 billion dollars in credit card debt alone.[3] What's more, the 2017 Financial Security Index survey by Bankrate.com revealed 29 percent of people aged eighteen to thirty-six had more credit card debt than emergency savings. Despite this crisis, only seventeen states in America require high school students to take a personal finance course before graduation. Yet becoming financially literate as a teen is associated with higher financial responsibility, such as better credit scores and lower delinquency rates, according to analysis by FINRA Investor Education Foundation.[4]

Experts believe financial literacy and associated behaviors should begin at home and during the preschool years. Unfortunately, many parents avoid talking with their family about money for fear of worrying their children or concern that they themselves are not financially fit. Modeling financial savvy, however, can be taught to and practiced by everyone, regardless of your financial history. Research finds that children with financial socialization experiences throughout childhood, such as holding savings accounts, are more likely as young adults to practice good financial habits and own financial assets other than bank accounts.[5]

Families who teach money skills throughout life will raise financially healthy children who have the confidence and skills to persevere through economic hardships and varying stages of life.

DID YOU KNOW?

Nearly one quarter of all millennials spend more than they earn. Only 33 percent have rainy day funds, a savings vehicle specifically for emergencies. And only four in ten are saving for retirement. This comes as no surprise, as only 22 percent of millennials participated in financial education in high school or college or through an employer.[6]

THE CHANGE
TEACH AND PRACTICE FINANCIAL RESPONSIBLITY.

PATH TO CHANGE   Get your family financially fit with the following tips:

OPT FOR CASH OVER CREDIT   With the growth in credit cards that earn hotel points and cash back, it has become easier and often preferred to use credit over cash. Unfortunately, credit cards make it easy for adults to overspend and difficult for children to understand the concept of budgeting. Young children may think the little magic card gets you everything you want! Opt to use paper money as often as possible, especially when your children are with you making a purchase, to practice good money habits. This will teach children how much things cost and how to spend money responsibly.

TEACH AGE-APPROPRIATE CONCEPTS   Learning to be financially responsible is a lifelong process that ideally begins during childhood. Focus on concepts most appropriate for your child's age to ensure that he or she will stay interested long enough to grasp the lesson. Also, repetition helps children understand money concepts in the same way it helps them learn how to ride a bike—so practice money skills often. Use the guidelines in the table to teach money concepts by age.

AGE	MONEY CONCEPTS
2 to 3 years	Money is used to purchase goods and services Coins versus bills
4 to 6 years	Cost of goods and services Spending money Simple budgeting Coin recognition Saving versus spending

6 to 8 years	Budgeting
	Concept of a bank
	Coupons and sales
	Saving for big-ticket items
	Philanthropy
9 to 12 years	Comparison of goods and pricing
	Debit and credit cards
	Budgeting
	Saving for the future, savings accounts
	Philanthropy
	Balancing accounts
13 to 17 years	Investment vehicles
	Budgeting with prepaid cards
	Work and payment
	Balancing accounts
	Credit reports
	Loans

SHOW MONEY DOESN'T GROW ON TREES   As adults, we've learned not to purchase everything we desire. Yet most children don't yearn for much because they receive many of the toys and gadgets they request. You can teach your family the value of money and budgeting by simply saying no to some requests for toys, clothes, or gadgets. Also, telling them, "We don't have the money for that this week" effectively models fiscal responsibility.

GIVE A MONETARY ALLOWANCE AND MONITOR THE MONEY   Provide a weekly monetary allowance to your children to teach them how to be savvy with their money. One dollar per year of age per week is often suggested, but choose an amount that fits within your financial limitations. Let children choose how to use their own money, but set guidelines to create learning opportunities and monitor how their money is used over time. For example, teach children how to save for the future by requiring them to set money aside weekly for college. Or help them understand the concept of budgeting by encouraging them to set money aside for a big-ticket item, such as a new bike.

MAKE SAVING A FAMILY AFFAIR   Learning how to save money is critical to achieve and maintain financial independence. Since most of us save money electronically through automatic deductions into 401(k)s or other investment accounts, however, the concept of saving has become intangible to children (and adults). Make saving a visible concept by using a simple savings jar and designating how the money will be used for the family. Choose things you will all enjoy, such as a trip to Disney World or a trampoline.

READ RELATABLE MONEY BOOKS   Incorporate books with lessons about money into reading time. Keep children engaged by choosing stories with characters that are interesting to your child. Young children may like the *Berenstain Bears' Trouble with Money* by Stan and Jan Berenstain or *Bunny Money* by Rosemary Wells. Older children may appreciate the Babysitters Club series by Ann Martin and *The Richest Man in Babylon* by George Clason. Centsables (www.centsables.com) is a financial education website for children featuring a series of fun comic books and activity books you can read online or as a PDF download. For teens, choose books you and your teen can read and discuss together, such as *Rich Dad, Poor Dad* by Robert Kiyosaki.

USE PREDESIGNED LESSONS   Instead of reinventing the wheel when teaching financial concepts, use lessons designed by financial education experts who specialize in teaching children of all ages. There are lessons for free and for purchase through online resources, such as www .econedlink.org, www.prosperity4kids.com, and www.consumerfinance.gov.

PLAY GAMES WITH MONEY   Family game night provides the perfect opportunity to teach monetary concepts in a fun, relatable fashion. Classics such as *Monopoly*, *Monopoly Jr.*, and *The Game of Life* teach concepts of investing, earning, and budgeting. You can also find fun online games for children and teens on www.kids.usa.gov/money and other financial sites recommended in this week's change.

PUSH THE BOUNDARIES

Life is either a daring adventure or nothing.
—HELEN KELLER

TAKING RISKS, TRYING new things, and testing our limits, whether we succeed or fail, creates a sense of invigoration, excitement, and adventure. Even more than adults, children need to experience these sensations to regulate fear, understand their own personal limits, manage frustration and anger, and build courage and confidence. Unfortunately, many of today's parents are raising kids in a culture of fear.

One study of six thousand *Slate* readers found "parents born in the 1970s were allowed to go to the playground alone and walk between 1 and 5 miles alone by second or third grade. When these people became parents they were more cautious with their own children, waiting until their kids were in fourth or fifth grade to just let them be outside by themselves."[1] Despite the shift to more restrictive parenting, data indicates that American children are safer from abduction, homicide, and getting hit by a car than they were thirty years ago.[2]

The trend in parenting, however well intentioned it may be, to over-protect our children from failure, disappointment, and the occasional booboo robs them of the chance to learn how to push themselves, reach for the stars, and experience the resulting happiness. According to psychologists who study human happiness, people who are truly happy believe taking risks beyond one's comfort zone is necessary for growth and development.[3]

For children, risk-taking play is the foundation for gaining skills needed to regulate themselves, not only in dangerous situations but also in everyday life, where balancing risk with reward is an ongoing task. Risk-taking play is defined as any type of play, often in the outdoors, where children face a reasonable risk of getting hurt. In Ellen Sandseter and Leif Kennair's famous paper "Children's Risky Play From an Evolutionary Perspective: The Anti-Phobic Effects of Thrilling Experiences," they define the six types of risk-taking play children need: heights, speed, separation/unsupervised play, handling dangerous tools or objects, and exposure to potentially dangerous elements.[4] This isn't to say you should hand your two-year-old a pair of garden shears, but research supports that your child will eventually need exposure to sharp objects in socially acceptable ways that test her limits—likely at a much earlier age than most modern, educated parents allow.

DID YOU KNOW?

Children may need to experience the thrill of heights (and even fall from a high place) to overcome a fear of heights. According to one longitudinal study, children without a fear of heights were more likely to have had falls that resulted in injury between the ages of five and nine.[5] Instead of restricting children from climbing high up in a tree or on a fence, let them determine how high they're comfortable climbing.

Limiting children, especially younger ones, from engaging in risk-taking play can be more detrimental in the long run. Children who aren't given opportunities to experience fear and manage risk will eventually find risks elsewhere. In Sandseter's work, she found that teenagers who couldn't feed their desire for risk and thrill in socially acceptable ways turn to much more reckless behavior, including drugs and alcohol.[6] Children of all ages, including teens, learn how to engage in healthy risk taking by mimicking their parents, so families can lower the chances of reckless behavior by incorporating healthy risk taking as early on as possible.

THE CHANGE
ALLOW YOUR KIDS TO TAKE HEALTHY RISKS.

PATH TO CHANGE   Your ability to embrace healthy risk taking enables your children to take risks and feel pride in their successful management of new experiences.[7] Use the following strategies to soar to new heights together:

DEFINE A "YES" SPACE   Children of all ages, from babies to middle schoolers, need to explore their world independently without constant oversight. Pay attention to how often you say, "No, don't go in there" or "No, that's not safe." Children must learn how to regulate themselves and make decisions without a watchful eye. Parents can create a safe space—or Yes Space—that allows them to roam and play freely without their parents saying no.[8] For older children, you can set boundaries in your neighborhood or a public space to facilitate independence and meet the need for separation/unsupervised play—one of Sandseter's six types of risks children need to experience. Saying yes is equally important for teenagers, especially when your child wants to try new skills or explore new places. Saying yes, within your financial limits, helps open the realm of possibility for your child to explore and push the boundaries of his existing talents and knowledge.

DO MEANINGFUL PROJECTS   Instead of forbidding your child to play with hammers, nails, or scissors, work together on a project that includes these types of tools. Including your child in meaningful projects is helpful to both the family and your child's development. Build a bookcase or a raised herb garden to practice using tools like hammers, drills, wrenches, handsaws, and other tools. Or do indoor projects with scissors, needles, and thread: make pillowcases or sew patches on torn pants.

MANAGE OR REMOVE HAZARDS   Letting children push their limits, especially physically, can mean greater risk of injury. Children will get bumps, bruises, and the occasional broken bone when given the freedom to explore their environment. You can manage injuries by removing hazards, such as unnoticeable sharp edges (such as barbed wire fencing) or structures that could collapse (such as partially fallen large trees). For very young children, scan their environment to remove dangerous hazards before independent play is available. For older children, make it a teaching opportunity to identify and discuss hazards together. Unfortunately, parents can't completely remove the hazards that teens commonly face, such as drugs, alcohol, high-speed driving, and unprotected sex. By encouraging teens to practice healthy risk taking you can reduce the temptation to engage in reckless behavior. Examples include auditioning for a school play, trying a new musical instrument, volunteering, scuba diving, or practicing a martial art.

LET THEM FAIL   For the most part, the failures our children experience when young are small in comparison to the challenges they may face as adults. When a child fails, it teaches him how to manage pride, overcome disappointment, and remain humble. It may break your heart as a parent, but letting your child fail makes him more resilient and teaches him how to succeed. Whether he builds a fort that falls down, loses at his favorite board game, or plays a baseball game without connecting with a single pitch, having you there to offer moral support, unconditional love, and encouragement provides security that helps your child go on to the next challenge. For older children, commiserating and sharing your own failures deepens your relationship, and builds trust, too!

TRY TOGETHER   Trying new things as a family is a perfect opportunity to help hesitant children learn how to venture beyond their comfort zone. Families can enjoy exhilarating activities, such as indoor rock climbing, or develop new skills or interests, such as painting or pottery. Share your emotions with your children about your experiences so they can see how you work through your own fears. Also, don't be surprised if your child doesn't want to participate. Many children learn through observation, so allowing them to say no while you test your own limits is still beneficial. With repetition, kids will start to surprise you with their own exploration of risk!

PUSH YOUR PARENTAL COMFORT ZONE   Think back to your own childhood. Were you allowed to play in the neighborhood alone, climb trees, or ride your bike to the corner store? These experiences helped define who you are and your own risk tolerance. They helped you to develop an internal compass for how to handle danger and risk. If your parents shielded you from these opportunities, you may have a very low risk tolerance. If you are a naturally protective parent, then start with small steps of relinquishing control. Give your child parameters that put you at ease, but don't limit her actions. For example, saying, "Remember, you have to climb back down the tree" is interpreted differently than "Don't climb too high." Finally, to get encouragement and reassurance, connect with friends and teachers who allow healthy risk taking.

BONUS

For parents of children six to twelve years old, visit outsideplay.ca for a fun tool, developed by child psychologists and researchers, to help parents get comfortable with their children's taking risks during outdoor play.

SKIP THE ADDITIVES

> Don't eat anything your great-grandmother
> wouldn't recognize as food.
> —MICHAEL POLLAN

THE MAJORITY OF packaged and premade foods contain food additives or added ingredients to preserve food, maintain appearance, and/or enhance flavor. Unfortunately, a growing body of evidence shows several commonly used food additives disrupt hormone levels, cause cancer and irreversible inflammation, alter mood and behavior, and induce developmental delays.[1] For example, butylated hydroxyanisole (BHA), an additive used to stabilize fats in foods such as chips, baked goods, and nuts, has been labeled a likely carcinogen by the National Toxicology Program. Further, animal studies show that BHA harms reproductive organs and alters hormone levels.[2] Another additive, propyl paraben, used as a preservative in foods such as baked goods, tortillas, and trail mixes, has been shown to lower testosterone and accelerate the growth of breast cancer cells and is linked to infertility in women.[3,4,5]

According to one study, at least a thousand food additives have made their way into our food supply without a thorough, objective evaluation of their safety by the FDA.[6] Food and nutrition industry expert Marion Nestle explains how this terrifying conundrum came about: "In 1997, the

FDA changed the approval process for food additives, shifting the burden of safety assessment from the FDA to food manufacturers themselves. Food manufacturers are now allowed to decide whether a new additive is generally regarded as safe (GRAS) for human consumption without even notifying the FDA."[7]

DID YOU KNOW?

The American Academy of Pediatrics (AAP) now recognizes that artificial food coloring and sodium benzoate, a common preservative used in food and medicines, both cause hyperactivity in children. For many years, the AAP publicly expressed skepticism about the link between additives and the behavior of children. But in 2008, Alison Schonwald, M.D., director of developmental and behavioral pediatrics at Children's Hospital in Boston, wrote a scientific review on behalf of the AAP in which she stated that the AAP was wrong in its original evaluation of the data. The AAP now recognizes that there is an abundance of evidence showing neurobehavioral toxicity is caused by commonly used food additives.[8]

Food in its natural state is loaded with vitamins, minerals, antioxidants, and macronutrients needed by your body for energy, to fight disease and infection, to balance hormones, and more. Poorly researched food additives added by manufacturers and grocers threaten your family's health in ways that are still being discovered.

Parents can have a major influence in shifting the family's food consumption to real food, free of harmful additives. For example, one study found children with parents who eat fruit and vegetables every day consume more fruits and vegetables than their peers with parents who do not eat produce daily.[9] By focusing on choosing real food without harmful additives, your family will enjoy better health and happiness, while also joining an ongoing movement of eating for good health.

THE CHANGE
CHOOSE WHOLE, REAL FOOD, WHILE AVOIDING UNHEALTHY ADDITIVES AND CHEMICALS.

PATH TO CHANGE   Avoiding food additives can seem like a daunting process if you try to revamp your pantry all at once. Use the following steps to navigate this change:

BUY WHOLE FOODS   Whole foods are fruits, vegetables, beans, nuts, seeds, whole grains, meat, poultry, seafood, cold-pressed vegetable and fruit oils (such as extra-virgin olive oil), and other foods that grow in the soil or on trees, or that come directly from animals, fish, or fowl, without any processing. They are consumed or cooked in their natural state or as you'd find them in nature. The more whole foods your family eats, the less likely you'll consume food additives, preservatives, and chemicals that can be harmful to your health.

Plan meals   Use the Seven-Day Weekly Menu Plan Worksheet in Part III: Tools and Resources to plan ahead for meals throughout the week. To make it even easier, create them electronically so that you can save completed weekly meal plans and repeat them often.

WHOLE FOODS

USE THE FOLLOWING suggestions to swap out processed food and add more whole foods to your family's nutritional plan.

PROCESSED FOOD	WHOLE FOOD ALTERNATIVE
Brownies	Dates, dried fruit
Boxed cereals	Rolled oats, steel-cut oats, buckwheat groats
Cheese crackers	Organic cheese
Cheese popcorn	Organic popcorn with nutritional yeast
Chicken nuggets	Chicken tenderloins (Dip in egg and coconut flakes and bake for a homemade nugget.)
Chocolate bars	Cacao nibs (and nuts)
French fries/tater tots	Roasted potatoes or homemade baked potato or sweet potato fries
Fruit Roll-Ups/ fruit snacks	Sliced whole fruit, unsweetened applesauce, dried fruit
Granola bars	Homemade trail mix containing nuts, seeds, and dried fruit
Potato chips	Kale chips

Focus on the perimeter of the store Whole foods are sold on the perimeter of the grocery store. This is where you'll find the produce section, the meat and seafood departments, and the dairy coolers. Shop the internal aisles for select items of whole grains, nuts, seeds, and frozen produce to complete your grocery trip.

READ LABELS   When searching for additive-free foods, skip the nutrition information and go straight to the list of ingredients. If you don't recognize an ingredient, it is likely a preservative or additive that could be harmful to your family's health. Keep in mind, food items with a long list of unfamiliar ingredients typically contain additives, so you may choose to avoid these all together.

BE DETECTIVES

Teach children how to search for additive-free, healthier packaged foods. Read labels with children and have them identify words they don't understand. To teach children how to search for additives on their own, use the Nutrition Detectives Program developed by Dr. David Katz, available online for free (www.davidkatzmd.com).

BEGIN WITH THE PANTRY OR FRIDGE   If your family is used to eating packaged foods, remove additives from your pantry or fridge by using the Pantry and Fridge Swap Worksheet in Part III: Tools and Resources to help find additive-free options. Start with the biggest offenders. For example, if your family loves packaged snacks, address these before moving on to other food categories. Every time you find a food item that contains additives, jot it down on the Pantry and Fridge Swap Worksheet to keep a running list of items for which you need additive-free alternatives. Search online for alternatives before going to the grocery store.

DINING OUT   Since most commercial condiments, packaged sauces, marinades, breads, cheese, and oils contain additives and preservatives, those served in restaurants likely do, too. This can make dining out without additives a bit more difficult, but not impossible.

Fast food Most fast-food restaurants use food products loaded with additives, chemicals, and other unhealthy ingredients. Recently, however, large restaurant chains have been committing to removing artificial ingredients from their foods. Check out the ingredient lists at your favorite fast-food joints to see if they've made similar efforts—if not, find a new venue.

Menu choices When in doubt about a restaurant's use of additives, encourage your family to choose fresh and simply prepared menu items. For example, order lightly seasoned or plain grilled meat or fish, roasted potatoes or other vegetables, and plain salads. To add dressing or flavor, ask your waiter for extra-virgin olive oil, vinegar, and lemon. Avoid fried foods and processed meat and cheeses, such as hot dogs, sausages, macaroni and cheese, and chicken nuggets. With or without additives, these foods are not good for your family's health.

Scratch kitchens Seek out restaurants known for making everything from scratch, to reduce the likelihood that additives are used. Search a restaurant's website for information about its philosophy on food and the ingredients it chooses to serve. Restaurants committed to serving real food will certainly let it be known because they have a competitive edge over other restaurants that use premade or precooked foods.

INSPIRE CHANGE AT SCHOOL OR DAY CARE Work with schools and day cares to improve nutrition by requesting salad bars, connecting schools with local farms, or incorporating fun into a traditional nutrition curriculum. In one study, adding salad bars to school cafeterias increased the amount and variety of fruits and vegetables consumed by students.[11] Other studies show that educating children about nutrition, additives, and food labels enhances their ability to distinguish more healthful from less healthful food.[12] Use the resources found on the National Farm to School website (www.farmtoschool.org) to get started.

SPREAD KINDNESS

No act of kindness, no matter how small,
is ever wasted.

—Aesop

THERE'S NO DENYING that being kind to others is the *right* thing to do. There is hard evidence, however, that being kind is also good for your health. Kindness has been shown to lower blood pressure, reduce pain, boost joyfulness, improve healing, and increase acceptance by peers (that is, popularity).

When an individual performs a kind act for us, such as holding the door or giving us their seat on the subway, these acts do not go unnoticed. As the recipient, we typically offer gratitude or even reciprocity when possible. The kind person experiences instant satisfaction and a psychological boost—benefits shown to improve joyfulness and engagement in life. In one randomized controlled study, university students who performed five random acts of kindness each day for one week had significantly higher positive emotions and better academic engagement than a control group.[1]

Helping others also increases oxytocin, a neurotransmitter associated with improved social bonds and better relationships. In fact, one controlled study of children aged nine to eleven across nineteen different classrooms showed performing acts of kindness not only increased life satisfaction and happiness of the children doing the acts, but it also boosted their popularity and acceptance by peers.[2] And developing stronger friendships offers many benefits to our children, as people with stronger relationships throughout life tend to be happier overall.[3]

For decades, Dr. Stephen G. Post, professor of family, population, and preventative medicine at Stonybrook University, has been studying the health benefits associated with helping others. He has found a growing body of research that shows individuals suffering from chronic pain and debilitating conditions, such as MS, experience psychological and physical improvements when they volunteer to provide emotional support to other people with similar conditions.[4,5] Fortunately, many experts in kindness, including author and researcher Dr. Sonja Lyubomirsky and Jeannette Maré, founder of the kindness-focused nonprofit Ben's Bells (www.bensbells.org), believe kindness is a skill that can be acquired, taught, and strengthened with direct guidance and intentional activities. And according to the work of the Harvard Making Caring Common Project, parents have a key role in raising children who prioritize kindness ahead of other important values, such as achievement. The more your family sets intentions to be kind and practices kindness, the more natural and unconscious this behavior becomes.

DID YOU KNOW?

Oxytocin, the neurotransmitter released during acts of kindness, reduces inflammation in the human body.[6] Inflammation is a key factor associated with common cardiovascular conditions such as atherosclerosis and heart disease.[7] Studies show people with chronic pain, cardiac trouble, and inflammatory conditions who perform kind acts for others also start to experience improvements in their mental and physical health.

THE CHANGE
TEACH KINDNESS AND PRACTICE INTENTIONAL KINDNESS DAILY.

PATH TO CHANGE   Research on kindness finds that people who explicitly set out to be kind each day and seek out opportunities to be kind experience improvements in their health and happiness. An added benefit is that spreading kindness is contagious, so your efforts are exponential in creating a more positive world. Use the following tips to flex your family's kindness muscles:

MONITOR YOUR KINDNESS   Your family likely already performs acts of kindness each day. Researchers suggest that people experience positive benefits from simply tracking the kind acts they receive and the kind acts they perform. Have family members track the acts of kindness performed by themselves and by others for them over the course of a week. Use the Kind Acts Tracking Worksheet found in Part III: Tools and Resources. To deepen the experience, speak with your family about how they felt when someone was kind to them and what they noticed about others after they were kind.

CELEBRATE KINDNESS WITHOUT REWARDS   It is common for parents to reward children when they achieve high marks in school or success in sports. Although providing rewards may seem to motivate children to perform specific behaviors (such as being kind) in the short term, research finds that when the rewards are no longer offered, these children are less likely to perform selfless acts of kindness.[8,9] Offering praise and compliments to your children for being kind instead of material rewards is more effective for encouraging them to continue their behavior. Studies show when mothers praise their child's good deeds, the children are more likely to perform prosocial behaviors or act in a way that is helpful and positive toward other people.[10,11]

BE KIND TO STRANGERS   Being kind to those we know within our inner circle is one way we strengthen our relationships. When it comes to strangers, however, kindness may not be as free flowing. Although young children are taught to not talk to strangers, eventually we expect children to respect other adults rather than fear them. You can help older children learn how to be kind to bus drivers, cashiers, barbers, and random children on the playground by helping them find common ground with them and by being friendly. For example, if a cashier is wearing a shirt for a baseball team, point it out to your son who loves baseball. This may encourage him to be friendly by striking up a casual conversation with the cashier. And of course, modeling to children that you are kind and appreciative of people who provide services to you and your family—such as bank tellers, school custodians, and mailmen—goes a long way in terms of teaching them to be kind to others.

DO KIND ACTS   Increase your family's interest in performing kind acts for others by choosing activities that align with their passions. Family members with musical talents, for example, can provide free concerts for residents at nearby nursing homes. Artistic family members might donate their artwork to local police and fire department personnel. Talk together as a family about the kind acts you'd like to perform for friends, neighbors, family, or other people in need, such as sick children or aging adults. Choose a day each week or every month to perform acts of kindness anonymously.

CONSIDER OTHERS' FEELINGS   Empathetic people are more inclined to demonstrate kindness because they can relate more easily to others. It is developmentally normal for young children to be focused on themselves, but with constant guidance from caregivers, a child can learn how to be empathetic. You can encourage empathy by consistently asking children questions, such as, "How would you feel if [fill in the blank] happened to you?" and having them explain how their actions impact others. Role-playing is also an effective way to teach and grow empathy in individuals. In one study, medical students developed greater empathy toward the elderly after a role-playing exercise. They had to wear goggles covered with tape to experience diminished vision and heavy rubber gloves to simulate decreased motor function.[12]

PRACTICE CARING   Like other skills, kindness and caring for others take practice. Children can deepen skills by taking responsibility for inanimate objects, such as toys, clothes, and the home, or by caring for pets. Age-appropriate chores give children a sense of ownership and pride in caring for something other than themselves. While having your child feed the fish every day or let the dog out to relieve herself may seem trivial, these acts are great practice in the art of kindness and caring. As children get older, continue to expand their responsibilities. For example, have driving-aged teenagers learn to wash the car, fill up the gas tank, and take it in for an oil change.

FULFILL OBLIGATIONS   You've likely experienced a situation where you committed to something, such as running in a charity run or hosting a holiday gathering, but as the event grew closer, you had second thoughts and hoped you could cancel. Your children have likely experienced the same situation. If avoiding obligations is going to hurt someone's feelings or cause a team to forfeit because of too few players, however, then allowing kids to back out sends them the signal that their interests are more important than the collective interests of others. You can use these experiences as learning opportunities to teach empathy as it relates to keeping our commitments. Of course, in cases where a child is feeling sick or overwhelmed, then canceling commitments is certainly warranted.

SILENCE THE NOISE

Silence is the sleep that nourishes wisdom.
—FRANCIS BACON

FROM THE ALARM that wakes us in the morning to the noise machine that lulls us to sleep at night, unless we seek silence, most of us are surrounded by noise all day, every day. Despite research linking noise to hypertension, increased incidence of diabetes, disordered sleep, and high stress, noise is often overlooked as a health risk factor.[1] Children are even more vulnerable to the effects of noise. Studies show chronic exposure impedes reading comprehension, memory, and attention, and is associated with cognitive impairment and emotional symptoms.[2,3,4]

Though noise pollution from involuntary sources may be higher in cities and near airports or major roadways, noise pollution from voluntary exposures, such as personal electronic devices, loud music, and background noise from the television, is also associated with negative effects. For example, background noise from the television has been linked to lower sustained attention during playtime, lower-quality parent-child interactions, and reduced performance on cognitive tasks.[5,6]

Silence, on the other hand, has the power to lower heart rate and blood pressure, even more than calming music.[8] Parents accustomed to waking in the wee hours of the morning, before the family rises, know firsthand about the amazing power of silence. Your thoughts are more organized, and you can concentrate and focus much better than when the sounds of life erupt. A fascinating animal study found that mice exposed to two hours of silence each day had higher levels of new brain cells than those without exposure to silence.[9]

Modern life is so loud and saturated with noise that when we are exposed to silence, it can be deafening. It can stir up unexpected emotions such as anxiety, stress, and worry. Families who seek ways to embrace silence regularly, however, can move through silence-inducing emotions and allow the benefits of silence to unfold, such as stilling the mind, calming the heart, and allowing the brain to rest and rejuvenate.

THE CHANGE
INCORPORATE SILENCE INTO EACH DAY.

PATH TO CHANGE Use the following tips to embrace silence and to teach children how to use silence as a way to quiet the mind and body:

TAKE A SIESTA Don't stop daily quiet time just because your children have aged out of preschool. Instead, schedule a period of quiet and rest in the afternoons, whenever possible. Refrain from turning on music or using devices to entertain family members; instead, encourage everyone to embrace the silence. The duration of quiet time, whether ten minutes or thirty, is not as important as creating a ritual, so that all family members look forward to and rely on resetting through silence. When it is difficult to stick with your quiet time ritual, remind yourself of the people in the Mediterranean and southern Europe who have made afternoon siestas a ritual for hundreds if not thousands of years.

TAKE MOMENTS OF SILENCE Schools often hold a moment of silence each day for quiet reflection, prayer, breath, or meditation. Incorporate similar moments of silence in your family life. Find natural times to take moments of silence each day, such as before you begin a meal, in the car before you head off to school or work, or in the evenings after dinner. Learning how to find silence in the middle of chaos is a skill your family will greatly benefit from for the long term.

CHOOSE SILENT ACTIVITIES Traditional family activities, such as playing sports, board games, or watching movies, can be especially noisy. Incorporate more time for silent activities into your family routine. For example, use tips from Week 18, Explore Nature, to spend more time in nature together, or Week 12, Just Breathe, to find time for meditating and deep breathing. Other ideas for silent activities include reading, playing card games, molding Play-Doh, building models, yoga, and arts and crafts. Encourage children of all ages to find silent activities that bring them joy.

SPEND TIME IN QUIET PLACES   We have become accustomed to loud, busy places and lots of noise wherever we go. This is especially true for those of us who live in urban or suburban areas. Instead of choosing noisy spaces, find quiet areas to enjoy time with friends and family, to do homework, or to relax. The more exposure your family has to quiet places, the better they will be at being contentedly in silence, especially when it's necessary, such as at a funeral or a wedding or during a presentation.

QUIET THE HOUSE BEFORE BED   After dinner and before bedtime can often be loud, with noise from the television, music, or video games. Schedule a couple of nights each week in which the house becomes quiet before bedtime instead. Turn the lights down to stimulate melatonin production for better sleep, and encourage your family to do quiet activities together or independently, such as reading, coloring, or, if you live in a quiet area, going outside and listening to the sounds of nature.

CREATE A QUIETER HOME   Fortunately, the availability of consumer products designed to reduce the amount of audible noise continues to grow. For the noisiest rooms, use sound-blocking curtains, thicker area rugs, and solid doors to limit noise from both outside and within the home. If your appliances are loud and noisy, consider purchasing newer models designed to disseminate less noise. If you need to replace windows, consider spending more for sound-insulating panes. Adding insulation to attics and gaps in outside walls helps too. Finally, purchase a set of high-quality noise-canceling headphones that family members can share (or purchase each member their own set if you can afford to). These headphones prove useful both in the home and on trips because they allow family members to partake in different activities without bothering one another.

GIVE BACK

If you can't feed a hundred people, then feed just one.
—Mother Teresa

SPREADING GOOD THROUGH volunteering and philanthropy benefits your community and our society at large. And it benefits you as well. According to research, altruistic adults report higher life satisfaction, well-being, and happiness.[1] Giving your time or money to a nonprofit or a religious or political organization for a cause you believe in provides a deeper sense of purpose and stronger connection to your world.

Volunteering is also associated with improved physical health, especially as you age. For example, one study showed older adults who volunteered at least two hundred hours in the past twelve months had lower blood pressure than adults who volunteered fewer hours. What's more, the adults who donated more time also reported improved well-being and increased physical activity.[2] Philanthropic activities naturally boost our happiness—an emotion that lowers our stress levels and improves our immune response.[3] In fact, people with chronic diseases who donate their time report a more positive outlook on life and lower levels of depression.[4] Although volunteering takes time and effort, the benefits are well worth it, especially considering research shows that people who volunteer are more likely to live longer and enjoy a higher quality of life, regardless of physical health.[5]

Skeptics question whether the health benefits of volunteering also apply to children, since volunteering commitments are not driven by the child's intrinsic motivation, but rather by the influence of parents, schools, or religious groups. Research refutes these concerns and shows children who volunteer have higher self-esteem, better self-confidence, improved academic performance, lower engagement in risky behaviors, and better health outcomes.[6,7,8] Further, teens who participate in service learning projects, through school or otherwise, have a stronger work ethic and deeper understanding of morality.[9]

Raising charitable children begins at home and can start as early as preschool age. A 2016 report titled the "Tradition of Giving" by the Indiana University Lilly Family School of Philanthropy found that parents and grandparents who volunteer or donate money are more likely to have children who do the same. Using data from an ongoing study of eight thousand families, researchers found that families who valued gener-osity passed this virtue on to future generations. And when children are allowed to pursue their own personal philanthropic interests as they grow into adolescents, they are more likely to continue volunteering and donating into adulthood.[10]

DID YOU KNOW?

Research shows that young children exhibit more happi-ness when giving to others. In one study, toddlers were given a set of treats to either enjoy themselves or share with treat-loving puppets they met during the experiment. Researchers measured the emotional response of the tod-dlers when they gave the treats away and when they con-sumed them personally. Toddlers did not exhibit aversion to giving, but instead showed more happiness when they gave the treats away.[11]

THE CHANGE
VOLUNTEER AND GIVE BACK.

PATH TO CHANGE   Many parents already feel stretched thin from managing work and family, but volunteering and charitable giving need not be an intensive commitment to be beneficial. Use the following recommendations to find ways your family can become more involved in giving back to the world.

BE A ROLE MODEL   Volunteering and charitable acts are particularly dependent on parental influence. For example, a national survey of 3,178 American youth revealed that children from families with at least one volunteering parent are almost two times more likely to volunteer and nearly three times more likely to volunteer on a regular basis compared with children from nonvolunteering families.[12] Find a volunteer opportunity that meets your time limitations, whether you can commit to two hours per year or two hours per month—there are loads of options available. Select a cause for which you care deeply to increase psychological fulfillment and the likelihood that you will continue volunteering.

TALK ABOUT GIVING   Talking to children regularly about charitable giving sets the stage for children to donate, too. A study by Lilly School of Philanthropy at Indiana University found 57 percent of children donated money to charity over multiple years when parents discussed charitable giving with them, as opposed to only 13 percent of children whose parents never spoke about giving.[13] You can help children understand the value of giving by sharing why and how your family gives to others. Offering explanations beyond "it is the right thing to do" provides context for children and tangible reasons for giving. For example, explain to children how money donated to a family in need may be used for food and clothing, so they get enough to eat and can learn, play, and perform at school and work.

FAMILY GIVING PROJECT   Carol Weisman, international volunteering expert and author of *Raising Charitable Children*, suggests connecting charitable discussions with action. For example, each holiday season Weisman brings her family together to discuss and choose a single philanthropic cause for the upcoming year. One year, familial concerns about health insurance led to the decision to sponsor one year of health insurance for a single mom with an asthmatic child.[14] You can apply a similar approach by choosing a cause that interests your family and spending the year finding ways to donate money or goods in support of the cause you have selected.

CHARITABLE GIVING BEYOND MONEY   Expand your charitable giving to include donations of goods and gifts, as well. By collecting and donating tangible items, young children who do not yet understand the concept of money are better able to participate in and benefit from charitable giving efforts.

<u>Goods</u>   Charities and nonprofits often need supplies and goods for their constituents. Your family can donate shelf-stable food items to a local food pantry, toys and books to a children's hospital, or clothes to a homeless shelter. Turn the act of providing goods to charity into a service project by collecting items from extended family members, classmates, and neighbors, too.

<u>Giving trees</u>   Buying anonymous gifts for others provides a unique opportunity for your family to practice giving without the expectation of getting anything in return. During the holiday season, many public libraries and civic organizations host giving trees where local families volunteer to purchase holiday gifts that have been requested by families in need. Children can participate in the gift selection, wrapping, and delivery of the gifts for a complete selfless experience of bringing joy to others.

<u>Homemade gifts</u>   Homemade gifts can be a special delight for those who otherwise receive only impersonal, store-bought items. As a family, you can bake cookies and deliver them to local police stations and fire

departments. Or you can create pictures or cards for residents of a local nursing home. Sometimes the simplest acts with a unique personal touch can bring the most joy to others.

VOLUNTEER TOGETHER   Volunteering as a family allows you to give to an organization while also spending quality time together as a family. You are more likely to create a successful volunteer experience if you choose age-appropriate volunteer opportunities. For example, bringing young children to serve food at a soup kitchen in the inner city might not be as rewarding or meaningful as collecting books and clothing to donate, or planting trees at a nearby park.

Move for a cause   There are athletic-based charity fundraisers happening all over the world. Find options you can participate in together as a family, such as walks, runs, and cycling events. Some charities have added kid-friendly versions of their larger athletic events, such as 1Ks or relay races, to encourage family participation. Find a nonprofit organization you care about and look for athletic events that help to raise awareness and money for their cause.

Get away   Families who love to travel can combine travel with volunteering through a volunteering vacation, also known as "voluntourism." There are many websites that provide information about different volunteer programs around the globe; most include a family volunteering section, too. Check out www.projects-abroad.org and www.globalfamilytravels .com. Or, if volunteering while traveling doesn't interest your family, you can check out www.packforapurpose.org to find nonprofits and charities in various countries that need supplies your family can collect, pack, and deliver while on your trip.

ENJOY HEALTHY FATS

Sugar, not fat, is the real villain that steals
our health and sabotages our waistlines.
—DR. MARK HYMAN

FOR DECADES, DIETARY fat was the villain of disease. Although recent research has debunked the myth that dietary fat is bad for your health, the low-fat philosophy still plagues America's eating habits. Yet dietary fat is actually vital to optimal health and many physiological functions.

Your body uses fat as a source of energy between meals. It enables your body to absorb fat-soluble vitamins A, D, E, and K, transporting them from your digestive system to your cells. Fat makes up the membranes protecting your cells, giving them fluidity and flexibility. It also manages the movement of critical substances in and out of your cells and has a role in gene expression.

That said, not all fat is created equal. Trans fat, manufactured by the food industry and found in many processed foods, causes heart disease and should be avoided. Good fats, such as monounsaturated and poly-unsaturated fats, including omega-3 and omega-6, however, contribute to good health.

UNDERSTAND YOUR GOOD FATS

SOME FATS OFFER unique benefits to our health.

+ MONOUNSATURATED FAT (MUFA):
Found in olive oil, avocados, and nuts, this type of fat benefits your heart and brain and even your body's ability to balance blood sugar.

+ POLYUNSATURATED FAT (PUFA):
Found primarily in nuts, seeds, and other plant foods, these fats are pre-cursors of substances vital to blood vessel constriction, blood coagulation, and immune system mediation. Two essential PUFAs that must be consumed through the diet are:

+ OMEGA-3 FATTY ACIDS: These fats elicit an anti-inflammatory immune response in your body. Research shows omega-3 fats, specifically the active forms known as DHA and EPA, improve heart and brain health through mechanisms such as improved blood flow and reduced coagulation of proteins. The Western diet is significantly lacking in these critical fatty acids. See Week 31, Go Fish, for tips on boosting intake.

+ OMEGA-6 FATTY ACIDS: Though still necessary for good health, these fats elicit an opposing, pro-inflammatory immune response in the body.[1] Whole foods rich in omega-6 fats offer protective health benefits and contain other vital nutrients, such as magnesium and vitamin E.[2] But oils extracted from these foods (such as sunflower oil) are chemically unstable and become easily oxidized when exposed to heat or air. Oxidized fat causes lesions in arteries and results in chronic inflammation, which leads to many types of disease. What's more, when consumed in excess, omega-6 fats inhibit conversion of omega-3 fats from ALA (the type found in plants) to EPA and DHA.[3,4]

+ SATURATED FAT: This category of fat is no longer linked to heart disease as it once was. Saturated fat contributes to an increase in HDL (protective "good" cholesterol) and lowers triglycerides. It produces larger, fluffier LDL cholesterol par-ticles that are less likely to damage arterial walls or cause a heart attack.[5,6,7,8,9] But quality of saturated fat matters, too. Of the five types of saturated fatty acids, some are inflammatory, while others are neutral in the body.

Unfortunately, the diets of most Americans are lacking in healthy fat. Packaged and prepared foods are staples, but these typically contain unhealthy fats because they're cheaper and more shelf stable. Products marketed to children are no different. The typical lunchbox often contains excessive amounts of less-healthy omega-6 rich oils, such as corn oil, soybean oil, safflower oil, and sunflower oil.

THE CHANGE
BOOST HEALTHY FAT INTAKE AND DECREASE UNHEALTHY FATS.

PATH TO CHANGE   Healthy fats are delicious and can be enjoyed in a variety of forms:

GET AN OIL CHANGE   Changing to healthy cooking oils is a surefire way to boost your family's intake of healthy fats and reduce consumption of unhealthy ones. Oils should be used for the cooking method most appropriate to the oil's heat tolerance and individual "smoke point." The smoke point is the specific temperature at which the oil starts to oxidize and its molecular structure changes, making the oil inflammatory and unhealthy. The higher the smoke point, the higher the temperature the oil can withstand. Upgrade your oils using the Recommended Oils by Use guide on the following page.

DID YOU KNOW?

The processing method can cause an oil to be more or less healthy. Many oils are produced by using extreme heat or by using heat and the chemical hexane. Heat can degrade the flavor, nutritional value, and color of the oil; hexane in large quantities is dangerous to our health.

Unrefined oils, however, are richer in nutrients, more robust, and true to their natural flavors. Cold-pressed oil uses a chemical-free process to extract oils from nuts or seeds by crushing them at very low heat, no higher than 120°F (50°C).

RECOMMENDED OILS BY USE

TYPE OF OIL	COOKING	MAX HEAT	BAKING	DRESSINGS	NOTES
Algae oil	✓	High			Surprisingly, has no fishy taste and is a source of active omega-3 fats (DHA).
Avocado oil	✓	High	✓		
Canola oil*	✓	High			Cold-pressed *only*; most canola oil is refined and extracted using hexane.
Coconut oil	✓	Medium to High	✓		Unrefined is best but has coconut flavor; use refined to avoid coconut flavor, though it's not as healthy.
Hemp seed oil				✓	
Flaxseed oil				✓	
Macadamia nut oil				✓	
Extra-virgin olive oil	✓	Low to Medium	✓	✓	Cold-pressed is best.

CONTINUES...

TYPE OF OIL	COOKING	MAX HEAT	BAKING	DRESSINGS	NOTES
Red Palm Oil	✓	High	✓		Unrefined *only*; will change color of food due to natural red color
Sesame Oil		Low		✓	Cold-pressed only; use sparingly
Walnut Oil				✓	

REDUCE INTAKE OF THESE OILS:

High in omega-6 fats, yet low in omega-3 fats, these oils are typically highly refined, thereby making them less stable and easily oxidized—or more inflammatory. Consume the whole food instead of oils from these foods.

+ **CORN OIL**

+ **SOYBEAN OIL**

+ **COTTONSEED OIL**

+ **SUNFLOWER OIL**

+ **SAFFLOWER OIL**

Expeller-pressing is a chemical-free process that extracts oil from nuts or seeds by crushing them with extreme pressure at various temperatures. Although the expeller-pressed oils are not treated with hexane during the expeller pressing process, note that they may be treated with hexane afterward to extract more of the remaining oil.

When you shop for oils, look for those that are unrefined, cold-pressed, or expeller-pressed.

Sautéing/pan frying Contrary to popular practice, not all oil is appropriate for high-heat cooking. For example, because of its prevalence in our culture, extra-virgin olive oil is commonly used with heat that is too high for safe consumption. If you overheat oil, you will see it smoking in the pan and notice a change in smell. When this happens, dump the oil, wipe the pan, and start with fresh oil on a lower heat setting.

Baking Any oil that can be heated on the stovetop can also be used in baking. Coconut oil has gained much popularity recently and for good reason. Though it is a saturated fat, coconut oil is high in lauric acid, an anti-inflammatory compound, and is used by the body as energy more quickly than other fats. Avocado oil has minimal flavor and can easily be used in baking, though it is more expensive than other baking oils. Extra-virgin olive oil has a stronger flavor and usually works best in more savory baked goods. Finally, unrefined red palm oil has a slightly sweet buttery flavor and is loaded with many antioxidants and vitamins. That said, not all palm oil is created equal. Be sure to choose unrefined, sustainably cultivated red palm oil that maintains its red color—otherwise the oil has been highly processed and is missing most health benefits.

Dressings Store-bought salad dressings are often loaded with additives and unhealthy ingredients, especially poor-quality oils. Upgrade dressings for salads and vegetable dipping by adding in nutrient-dense oils. Flaxseed oil, one of the richest sources of plant-based omega-3 fat, has a nutty flavor and is also full of lignans, a polyphenol, or plant compound, associated with lower risk of breast cancer and heart disease. Other oils to consider include avocado oil, hemp seed oil, macadamia nut oil, sesame oil, walnut oil, and, of course, extra-virgin olive oil.

LOAD UP ON SEEDS   Many types of seeds are rich in healthy fats, protein, vitamins, and minerals. Plus, with the recent growth in nut allergies, seeds are a safe and healthy alternative for all children.

TYPE OF SEED	NUTRITIONAL BENEFITS	HOW TO EAT THEM
Chia	High in omega-3 fats and fiber; packed with calcium, magnesium, and phosphorus, all good for bone health	Atop salads and oatmeal; make a pudding or thicken soup
Pumpkin (with or without shells)	High in polyunsaturated fat and iron (23 percent of daily recommended value for adults), magnesium, copper, and zinc	Alone, in trail mix, atop salads or veggies
Sesame	Highly nutritious source of calcium, magnesium, iron, zinc, and manganese	Atop salads, stir-fry dishes, and cooked veggies; grind 5 parts sesame seeds with 1 part Celtic sea salt to create "gomashio," a salt alternative
Sunflower	Excellent source of monounsaturated fat, vitamin E, copper, selenium, and vitamin B1 (thiamine)	In trail mix or atop salads, or pureed to create sunbutter, a nut butter alternative

GO NUTS   Like seeds, nuts are also loaded with high-quality fats, protein, vitamins, and minerals. You can eat them alone or as part of trail mix. Other options include pureed into nut butter, atop salads and vegetable dishes, baked in desserts and muffins, soaked and strained into milk, or ground up and used as flour. Here are a few highly nutritious favorites:

TYPE OF NUT	NUTRITIONAL BENEFITS
Almonds	Quality source of monounsaturated fats; higher in calcium than other nuts, and high in vitamin E, riboflavin, manganese, magnesium, and phosphorus, with a little iron
Brazil nuts	Good source of polyunsaturated fats; plus, a serving has over 500 percent of the daily recommended value of selenium, a powerful antioxidant
Cashews	Great source of monounsaturated fats; loaded with copper, zinc, and magnesium; source of vitamin K and folate, two nutrients many of us don't get enough of
Hazelnuts	Good source of monounsaturated fats; contains magnesium, vitamin B6, and fiber
Hemp seeds (hemp hearts)	Highly nutritious seed that is actually a tiny nut from the hemp plant; exceptionally rich source of omega-3 fats and complete protein, containing all essential amino acids; packed with fiber and rich in magnesium, vitamin E, zinc, and iron
Pistachios	Source of potassium (to benefit blood pressure) and fiber
Macadamia	Slightly higher in saturated fat than other nuts, but a good source of monounsaturated fat; loaded with manganese, a mineral critical for bone health
Walnuts	Quality source of omega-3 fats; contains copper, magnesium, manganese, vitamin B6, and folate

SERVE FATTY FRUIT   Avocados and olives are actually fruits loaded with monounsaturated fat. Olives can be eaten alone or added to fish, casseroles, salads, and Mediterranean dishes. Avocados are the base for guacamole, but also make great additions to smoothies, salads, and creamy sauces.

READ LABELS   Most packaged food products rely on pro-inflammatory fats or omega-6 fats like soybean oil, corn oil, safflower oil, sunflower oil, corn oil, and peanut oil. Read the ingredients list and find products that contain healthier oils, such as coconut and extra-virgin olive oil.

CLEAN UP THE CHEMICALS

When it comes to profit over safety, profit usually wins.
—JAMES FRAZEE

YOUR FAMILY IS exposed to hundreds of chemicals every day. For the most part, your liver does an excellent job at detoxification and ensures that you excrete toxins through urine, sweat, and stool. Unfortunately, many chemicals absorbed through the skin, inhaled when sprayed, or consumed through oral exposure have proven to be toxic and detrimental to our health, yet they are still allowed in personal care products, household cleaning products, and more.

Personal care products, including sunscreens, lotions, hair products, and diaper creams, are of particular concern when it comes to chemicals. These substances are rubbed on your skin, a porous organ, and readily absorbed into your body. Given that the average person uses nine personal care products daily (teens use seventeen products daily), exposure to chemicals in these products is a concern. Unfortunately, according to the FDA, "with the exception of color additives and a few prohibited ingredients, a cosmetic manufacturer may use almost any raw material as a cosmetic ingredient and market the product without approval from the FDA."[1]

Nearly one in five cosmetics and personal care products contain preservatives known as formaldehyde releasers. These are chemicals that decompose slowly over time to form molecules of formaldehyde.[2] Both the U.S. government and the World Health Organization (WHO) have classified formaldehyde as carcinogenic when inhaled, and research shows that personal care products can release small amounts of formaldehyde into the air after they are applied.[3]

Triclosan or triclocarban is another chemical used in a variety of products, including antibacterial soap, body wash, deodorant, and toothpaste; it has been shown to disrupt hormones and cause muscle weakness and toxicity to the liver. In 2017, the FDA banned use of this ingredient in antibacterial soap, but it remains in other commonly used products, such as a top-selling toothpaste.[4]

Scientific evidence shows that reducing exposure to products containing toxic chemicals can reduce the toxic load in the body, thereby lowering the health risks associated with long-term exposure. In one study, researchers had one hundred adolescent girls refrain from using products containing three sources of endocrine-disrupting chemicals: phthalates, parabens, and phenol. They measured urinary concentration of these chemicals before stopping use of the products, and again three days after stopping, and found significant reductions in toxic load.[5] Families can reduce exposure to toxic chemicals by avoiding brands and products that use concerning ingredients.

DID YOU KNOW?

The European Union (EU) restricts the use of over 1,400 chemicals in personal care products, most of which are allowed in the United States. The EU's approach to chemical management, referred to as "better safe than sorry," is based on a policy called the precautionary principle.[6,7] Unlike in the United States, a chemical is restricted if there is any credible scientific evidence of danger to human health, even if scientific certainty is not established.

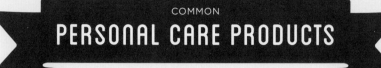

PERSONAL CARE PRODUCTS

USE THIS GUIDE to understand what to look for and avoid with common personal care products.

PERSONAL CARE PRODUCT	WHAT TO KNOW AND AVOID
Toothpaste	Choose brands without parabens, triclosan, or artificial colors, since residue of these toxic chemicals remains in the mouth after use.
Hair spray	Particles are easily inhaled and absorbed into the scalp. Many contain phthalates, phenol, and other concerning ingredients. Choose brands with plant fibers, such as Acacia Senegal Gum for staying power and essential oils for scent.
Nail polish	Many polishes contain formaldehyde, aluminum, and endocrine-disrupting plasticizers, such as phthalates. Choose those committed to using nontoxic ingredients, such as Acquarella, Piggy Paint, and Suncoat.
Face and body lotions (or butters)	Many have names that sound natural, such as "Honey Milk," but contain nasty ingredients, including fragrance, parabens, formaldehyde releasers, toxic surfactants, and more. Choose those with a list of recognizable ingredients, such as nut and plant oils, cocoa or shea butters, and essential oils for scent.
Shampoo and conditioner	Many contain parabens, polyethylene glycol (PEG) compounds, formaldehyde, allergy-causing surfactants, and other carcinogenic ingredients. Since residue absorbs into your scalp, it is best to choose organic brands or versions without harsh chemicals, fragrance, or preservatives.

THE CHANGE
CHOOSE PERSONAL CARE AND HOUSEHOLD CLEANING PRODUCTS THAT LOWER EXPOSURE TO TOXIC CHEMICALS.

PATH TO CHANGE   Lower your family's health risks associated with long-term exposure to toxic chemicals by having family members choose safer personal and household products:

UPGRADE PERSONAL CARE PRODUCTS   Chemicals found in personal care products do not require testing and are not regulated by the FDA. Find healthier products using the Environmental Working Group's Skin Deep database (www.ewg.org/skindeep), an online searchable tool that includes ratings and safety information for tens of thousands of skin care products. To get started, use the following tips:

USE SAFER SUNSCREEN   A growing body of research shows that many active ingredients in sunscreen pose potential health risks to your family. One of the most widely used UV filters, oxybenzone, is associated with higher levels of endometriosis in women, infertility in men, and increased levels of the chemical in breast milk.[8,9,10] The Environmental Working Group keeps an up-to-date list of the safest sunscreens, which can be found on their website at www.ewg.org. See Week 6, Befriend the Sun, for more information about safe sun exposure.

DID YOU KNOW?

One study by Duke University and the EWG found that women who had their nails painted with a polish that contained TPHP, an endocrine-disrupting hormone, had a sevenfold increase in the amount of TPHP in their bodies just ten to fourteen hours after application.[11]

GO FRAGRANCE-FREE The "fragrance" found in everything from perfume to household cleaners is made up of many different chemicals, some of which have been linked to allergies and hormone disruption. For example, phthalates found in fragrance help make scents stick to skin, but they are known endocrine disruptors and have been banned in cosmetics by the European Union.[12] Choose products with essential oils instead of fragrance for scent.

BUY NATURAL HOUSEHOLD CLEANERS The natural cleaning market has experienced explosive growth in the past few years, but many products still contain concerning chemicals due to lack of federal oversight. Further, manufacturers are not required by law to include an ingredient list on cleaning products. To be safe, choose brands that list ingredients on the package and opt for environmentally friendly certified green products. Or, better yet, make your own all-purpose cleaner using vinegar. Vinegar has been used as a disinfectant for thousands of years, and a recent study showed it has the power to kill mycobacteria, the bacteria that causes tuberculosis. Simply fill a spray bottle with white vinegar, and add 10 to 15 drops of essential oil, such as lemon, lavender, or mint, for a nicely scented DIY cleaning solution.

AVOID ANTIBACTERIAL OPTIONS According to the FDA, research does not demonstrate that antibacterial soaps are better at preventing illness than washing with plain soap and water. Avoid these products, which often contain toxic chemicals.

TAKE EXTREME MEASURES WITH CHILDREN'S PRODUCTS It takes a lot longer for babies and young children to metabolize toxic chemicals, because of their small size. Use as few products as possible with your youngest family members, and choose reputable natural brands, such as Beauty Counter and California Baby, that are recommended by the Environmental Working Group.

CHEMICALS TO AVOID IN PERSONAL CARE PRODUCTS

INGREDIENT	WHY IT'S BAD	WHERE IT'S FOUND
Benzalkonium chloride	Associated with severe skin, eye, and respiratory irritations and allergies; dangerous for people with asthma	Sunscreens, moisturizers
Benzophenone and derivatives	Possible human carcinogen and hormone disruptor	Nail polish, sunscreen
Boric acid and sodium borate	Can cause irritation to eyes and skin; possible hormone disruptor	Diaper creams
BHA and BHT	Hormone disruptors that may also alter DNA	Lipsticks, moisturizers, diaper creams
Coal-tar hair dyes and other coal-tar ingredients	Known carcinogen	Hair dye, shampoo
Ethanolamines (MEA/DEA/TEA)	Linked to allergies, skin toxicity, hormone disruption, and inhibited fetal development	Hair dyes, mascara, foundation, fragrances, sunscreens, dry cleaning solvents, paint, pharmaceuticals
Ethylenedi-aminetetraacetic acid (EDTA)	May be toxic to organs	Hair color, moisturizers
Formaldehyde	Linked to neurotoxicity and asthma	Shampoo, body wash, bubble bath
Formaldehyde releasers (Bronopol, DMDM hydantoin, diazolidinyl urea, imidzaolidinyl urea, and quaternium-15)	Known human allergen and skin toxicant; may be toxic to immune system	Shampoo, conditioner, bubble bath
Fragrance	Toxic to immune system and respiratory system and can cause allergies	Many personal care products
Hydroquinone	Linked to cancer, organ toxicity, and skin irritation	Skin-lightening creams

CONTINUES...

INGREDIENT	WHY IT'S BAD	WHERE IT'S FOUND
Lead acetate	Toxic to human reproductive system; possible human carcinogen	Men's hair dye
Methylisothi-azolinone and methylchloroiso-thiazolinone	Most common irritants and causes of skin allergies	Shampoo, conditioner, body wash
Oxybenzone	Linked to irritation and allergies and possible hormone disruptor	Sunscreen, moisturizer
Parabens (methyl-, isobutyl-, propyl-, and others)	Disrupts hormones	Shampoo, face cleanser, body wash, body lotion, foundation
Petroleum distillates	Possible human carcinogen; may be toxic to gastrointestinal system and liver	Mascara
Phthalates (DBP, DEHP, DEP, and others)	Disrupts endocrine system and may cause birth defects	Synthetic fragrance, nail polish, hairspray
Polyethylene glycol (PEG compounds)	Linked to cancer	Creams, sunscreen, shampoo
Resorcinol	Toxic to immune system and organs; potential hormone disruptor	Hair color, bleaching products
Retinyl palmitate and retinol (vita-min A)	May speed growth of tumors when used topically	Moisturizer, antiaging skincare
Sodium lauryl sulfate and sodium laureth sulfate (SLS and SLES)	Linked to skin irritation and allergies	Shampoo, body wash, bubble bath
Toluene	Toxic to immune system and can cause birth defects	Nail polish
Triclosan and triclocarban	Disrupts human reproductive systems	Liquid soap, soap bars, toothpaste, deodorant

Sources: Environmental Working Group, BeautyCounter.

CLEANING INGREDIENTS TO AVOID

INGREDIENT	WHY IT'S BAD
2-butoxyethanol (also ethylene glycol monobutyl ether and other glycol ethers)	Damages red blood cells and potentially causes anemia Creates air pollution that exceeds workplace limits Linked to impaired fertility, reproductive and developmental toxicity Considered a possible human carcinogen by EPA
Alkylphenolethoxyl-ates	Breaks down into alkylphenols—potent hormone disruptors widely detected in people and the environment Although E.U. and Canada banned them in cleaning supplies, U.S. has not Other terms: nonyl- and octylphenolethoxylates, or non- and octoxynols
Dye	Generic term that includes many ingredients, including toxic substances; best avoided
Ethanolamines	May contribute to the development of asthma May be carcinogenic or neurotoxic Variations: mono-, di-, and tri-ethanolamine
Fragrance	Can contain hundreds of untested chemicals, including toxic ingredients like phthalates and synthetic musks, both of which are hormone disruptors; known allergens
Pine or citrus oil	Forms carcinogenic formaldehyde if used on smoggy/high-ozone days
Quaternary ammonium compounds (quats)	Can contribute to development of asthma May lead to development of bacterial resistance to these and other germ-killing chemicals Also look out for: alkyl dimethyl benzyl ammonium chloride (ADBAC), benzalkonium chloride, and didecyl dimethyl benzyl ammonium chloride

GROW YOUR MIND

I have no special talents. I am merely inquisitive.
—ALBERT EINSTEIN

PARENTS OF OLDER children can certainly remember the adorable (and mildly irritating) phase when their child asked questions about everything. *Why is the sky blue? Why does it rain? Why is it hot today? Why are strawberries red?* It turns out that fostering curiosity and a love of learning, as young children demonstrate by their endless questioning, leads to a longer life of more success, happiness, and well-being.

Constantly learning new skills and building knowledge makes us more interesting, dynamic individuals and brings more joy to life. In fact, scientists discovered that satisfying one's curiosity releases dopamine, a neurotransmitter that lifts your spirits and makes you feel happy. Using magnetic resonance imaging (MRI), researchers also saw that satisfying curiosity activated the limbic reward system of the brain, indicating we take pleasure in learning new information that interests us.[1]

Developing new skills also keeps your mind sharp and your memory strong, especially into old age. In one study, researchers compared the minds of three groups of older adults who either (1) learned and practiced a cognitively demanding new skill, (2) engaged in nonintellectual social activities, or (3) pursued low-demand cognitive tasks with no social contact. After just three months, those who learned and practiced a new skill experienced cognitive improvements in episodic memory, visuospatial processing, and speed at which they performed mental tasks, compared to the other two groups.[2] Challenging your mind improves brain function and supports neurogenesis, a process in which new neurons and neural pathways are created in the brain, increasing intelligence.

Young children are naturally curious and have an innate desire to learn and master new skills. Sadly, the internal fire for knowledge tends to wane by third grade as outside social pressures take over. Like teachers, parents have the power to promote an ongoing interest in learning. For example, a multiyear study showed that children with parents who encouraged them to ask questions, exposed them regularly to new experiences, and promoted curiosity had both a stronger interest and higher achievement in science than peers whose parents did not promote curiosity.[3] Families that provide a supportive learning environment and make personal growth a priority can raise children who are happier and have a lifelong passion for knowledge.

THE CHANGE
PROMOTE CURIOSITY AND ENCOURAGE A LOVE OF LEARNING.

PATH TO CHANGE   Grow your mind and boost happiness by promoting curiosity and a love of learning using the following strategies:

LEARN TOGETHER   Schedule regular family outings to nature centers and zoos, science and art museums, cultural centers, or historical societies. Explore markets, bazaars, and even antique shops for a unique way of learning about art, history, and music.

BE EXPLORERS   Instead of visiting the same location each year for your family vacation, explore and discover the world together. Get travel books and maps, and encourage older children to plan your adventure. Throughout the year, get children involved in finding new destinations to visit on weekends.

BUILD ON YOUR FAMILY'S INTERESTS   It is easy to pique your children's curiosity when you focus on topics that already have their interest. In his book *Sparks: How Parents Can Ignite the Hidden Strengths of Teenagers*, Peter Benson explains that children are more motivated to learn when they've discovered their "sparks"—the activities and interests that light fire in their lives. If your child goes through a Spider-Man phase, visit a science museum or zoo to look at the spiders. Take out library books about different kinds of spiders, or build life-size spiderwebs together using yarn. The same goes for older children—if your child loves baseball, learn about the players that have made it to the Baseball Hall of Fame, take trips to different baseball fields, and look up different techniques for throwing and hitting the ball.

LEARN FROM EXPERTS   Most people naturally love to share their knowledge and skills, especially with children. It's fun to read about a topic that interests your child, but consider visiting an actual expert. For example, the next time your child asks, "How do you make shoes?" visit the local cobbler. As children get older, connecting with experts in various industries can be especially helpful for college applications and career exploration.

LOOK IT UP   With the advent of Google, there is virtually nothing your family can't find on the Internet. When you have a burning question or your child has one, take a minute to research together online. Show your child how to create an effective search on Google or other search engines. And show her how to find reputable sources for the answers. Children will also enjoy visiting a library and finding printed resources to satisfy their curiosities and questions.

STIMULATE CURIOSITY AT HOME   First, surrounding your children with books covering a range of genres and topics stimulates a love of learning. For younger children, add toys especially designed to stimulate curiosity, such as kinetic sand, magnetic blocks, and water toys that include different-size funnels, colorful pipes, and water wheels. For school-aged children, purchase binoculars, Little Bits and other circuit sets, vex robotics, butterfly or ant farms, laboratory play sets, telescopes, and woodworking kits.

ONLINE ACADEMIES   Introduce your children to free online schools such as Khan Academy (www.khanacademy.org), which offers access to novel teaching methods and online classrooms that cover a plethora of topics. That said, be sure to monitor screen activities for duration and age-appropriateness.

USE POSITIVE FEEDBACK RATHER THAN REWARDS   According to Dr. Carol Dweck, author of *The Growth Mindset*, praising hard work and effort cultivates a propensity for children to take on more challenges and learn from them, whereas praising children for their intelligence can lead to less enjoyment, lower persistence, and worse performance in an activity.[4] Instead of offering rewards, find ways to celebrate your child's curiosity and love of learning; for instance, hang their work on the walls, share their findings with grandparents and friends, and keep a journal to document the interesting things they've discovered.

MODEL A LOVE OF LEARNING   Make time to engage in learning opportunities that satisfy *your* curiosities and new interests, as well. For example, adults can go back to school for certifications and degrees and to take continuing education classes. If a new degree doesn't interest you, find local workshops or conferences that cover topics of interest. Parents who satisfy their internal interests to learn and grow can naturally pass a love of learning to their children.

BUILD
INNER STRENGTH

Do not judge me by my success; judge me by how
many times I fell down and got back up again.

—NELSON MANDELA

AS PARENTS, WE hope to protect our children from trauma, danger, and grief, and to watch them work through adversity to achieve success, whatever that may be in their eyes. But rather than raising them in a bubble, it turns out that helping our families build resiliency and grit may serve them best.

Resiliency protects people in times of trauma and sadness. Numerous studies show that resilient people have higher resistance to stress, lower rates of depression, and faster recovery after trauma such as cardio-vascular events—they aren't knocked down by experiences that might otherwise be deflating or unbearable.[1]

Resilient people are also able to adapt when faced with hardships and to persevere through adversity. Through years of studying high achievers, psychologist and author Angela Duckworth found that "grit," a term she used to describe resiliency as it relates to success, was more predictive of achievement than IQ, SAT scores, the prestige of the university attended, or top scores on military performance tests. Duckworth says that people "who are unusually resilient, hardworking and willing to continue in the face of difficulties, obstacles and even failures" are the most successful in life.[2] Having grit essentially increases a person's chances for achievement, despite setbacks.

Resiliency is also highly associated with longevity. One study evaluated the resiliency of adults aged sixty-five to one hundred and older, and found centenarians (people one hundred or older) to be the most resilient population. Further, people aged ninety-four to ninety-eight with the highest resiliency scores were 43 percent more likely to become centenarians than their less-resilient peers.[3] And it's highly likely that centenarians are enjoying these extra years, because people who are the most resilient also report greater happiness and more satisfaction in life.[4]

Experts find that we can develop resilience at any age. Building this quality in yourself and your family starts with having strong relationships and being part of a supportive community. Positive and meaningful relationships instill a sense of hope and optimism that is empowering when one is faced with a struggle or a stressor. Working together as a family to boost positivity, embrace gratitude and kindness, nurture your faith and cultural traditions, and take care of your health are the foremost activities associated with resiliency in both adults and children.

DID YOU KNOW?

A study that spanned forty years helped researchers discover why some children can persevere through extreme hardship while others cannot. In the famous Kauai Longitudinal study, 30 percent of "high risk" children developed into competent, confident, and caring adults, despite having grown up in families troubled by chronic poverty, perinatal stress, domestic violence, addiction, and mental illness. The study found that children who persevered may have done so because of the consistent nurturance they received throughout life from substitute caregivers, such as grandparents, extended family, peers, or other adults, whom they relied on for constant emotional support and counsel.[5]

THE CHANGE
ADOPT TOOLS AND PRACTICES THAT FOSTER RESILIENCE AND GRIT.

PATH TO CHANGE Strengthening your family's resolve won't happen overnight, but it is certainly possible with the adoption of behaviors highly associated with resiliency. Use the following suggestions to get started:

USE ADAPTIVE COPING STRATEGIES Psychologists suggest that taking specific actions to address the root problem of a stressor can be an effective coping strategy. For example, if your child is too tired in the afternoon to focus and enjoy school, teach her to prioritize more sleep or modify her lunch to sustain her energy. Other examples of using actions to cope include creating plans to address challenges or big projects, soliciting help from others, documenting pros and cons to think through decisions, and turning down requests when you are already busy. By regularly practicing and talking about ways to resolve problems with action, your family is less likely to resort to unhealthy coping strategies when overwhelmed or faced with setbacks and stress.

FOSTER OPTIMISM Staying positive is better for your health and can be taught and improved, even in adults. One study followed 135 adults over six years and discovered when optimists faced stress, they did not experience an elevation in cortisol (the stress hormone) in the same way their pessimistic peers did.[6] We can shift pessimistic mindsets by using language that reinforces setbacks (and success) as normal and temporary. Talk often about the power we have as individuals to overcome challenges and see them as opportunities rather than taking a powerless or defeated stance.

PRACTICE REFLECTION Resilient people still experience emotion; however, they tend to view failure objectively and evaluate themselves and the situation in order to accept it, learn from it, and move on. When faced with pain or challenges, start by acknowledging your feelings and think what could be done differently so history doesn't repeat itself. Take this same approach with your children by modeling how to reflect on failures and guiding them through their own reflective process. For example, if you accidentally yell at your child (it's okay—we all do sometimes), use it as an opportunity to admit your misstep and explain what you'll do to avoid yelling in the future.

PROMOTE HEALTHY RISK TAKING   Children who practice healthy risk taking are building resiliency. When your child is climbing trees or trying out for the school play, she is building problem-solving skills, courage, and self-esteem—experiences and character traits that strengthen resiliency and grit. The same goes for adults who push beyond their comfort zone and try new skills and activities—you are strengthening your confidence and ability to work through problems. Use the tips in Week 34, Push the Boundaries, to nudge yourself and your family out of their comfort zone and become more resilient!

COMPLIMENT EFFORT AND HARD WORK   In modern society, we have a natural tendency to celebrate successes rather than effort. For example, in school, children who achieve the best grades and make the honor roll receive awards, regardless of the effort put in to achieve those grades. Research shows that children who are praised for effort, however, are more inclined to try harder and persist longer than those who are praised for performance. Find ways for your family to celebrate hard work, not just success. Offering encouraging remarks to recognize hard work, determination, and effort may seem trite, but it reinforces to children that persistence pays off.

WHEN QUITTING IS HEALTHY   Modern society has led us to believe that quitting is horrible and should be avoided at all costs. Resiliency expert Angela Duckworth, however, states that quitting might be the best course of action in some instances. Although quitting when times get tough or hardship is faced seems to negate the fostering of resiliency, Duckworth's research on grit finds that if passion and interest are lost, then quitting may be the best course of action. Since childhood is a time for exploration of interests, sports, and hobbies, you may find your children are more apt to quit things they find uninteresting. Discuss quitting with your children, and find a balance that allows them to continue exploration without the fear of quitting.

PRACTICE WITH PASSION   It is much easier to tolerate setbacks and failures when you are passionate and excited about the project, task, or activity. Help your family practice resiliency by nurturing their passions. As a person grows his skills in a particular extracurricular activity, sport, or subject at school, it's expected he will face challenges and stumbling blocks. These experiences naturally develop confidence, strength, and resiliency, and provide references to inspire perseverance in future times of hardship.

BUILD SUPPORTIVE RELATIONSHIPS   Having strong, supportive relationships provides us with the comfort of security and safety needed for resiliency. Take time to strengthen your own relationships with your spouse, your family, and close friends. And help children develop relationships built on mutual respect, love, and support. Use tips from Week 16, Be a Good Friend, to support your family in building a community of strong relationships on which to rely in both good and tough times.

GET INSPIRED   People of all ages can be inspired when hearing stories about others who have faced adversity and persevered. Seek out books, films, and other media that interest your family and model resiliency and grit. Young children will love *Horton Hears a Who* by Dr. Seuss and *The Most Magnificent Thing* by Ashley Spires. Tweens and teens may enjoy the Hunger Games trilogy by Suzanne Collins and *A Long Walk to Water* by Linda Sue Park. Resiliency is infectious, and parents can benefit from reading true stories of resiliency to boost their own strength and determination, too.

GO ORGANIC

Let food be thy medicine and medicine be thy food.
—Hippocrates

CONSUMERS AND EXPERTS alike cite numerous reasons for choosing
organic over conventional food, such as better taste, improved nutrition, and the fact that it is better for our environment. Though some of
these arguments are subjective and perhaps inconsistent across sources,
research provides unwavering proof that exposure to pesticides is detrimental to your family's health. And unless your family lives or works
close to a farm, food is considered the primary pathway of pesticide
exposure, especially in children.

Conventional farming uses hundreds of synthetic pesticides and fertilizers throughout the growing process to battle insect infestations and
ensure crop yields. These chemicals can seep into plant matter and
remain on skins of vegetables and fruit, even after they've been washed.
Research has linked several of these commonly used chemicals to cancer
and other chronic health issues, including abnormal neural development,
asthma, disruption of fetal growth, and endocrine disruption. For example, glyphosate (the most widely used herbicide worldwide, also known

as Roundup) has been studied extensively for its link to cancer. In March 2015, the WHO's International Agency of Research on Cancer (IARC) concluded that glyphosate is a probable human carcinogen. Further, in March 2017, California's Office of Environmental Health Hazard Assessment (OEHHA) announced that glyphosate would be added to the list of chemicals known to cause cancer via Proposition 65, which passed a law requiring that special warnings be placed on products containing harmful chemicals.[1] Yet glyphosate continues to be allowed by the Environmental Protection Agency (EPA) in conventional farming practices.

DID YOU KNOW?

Just switching from conventional produce to organic produce can significantly reduce your family's exposure to pesticides. In a study of twenty-three school children, researchers analyzed urine before and after dietary changes were implemented and measured significantly higher levels of toxic chemicals when conventional produce was consumed rather than organic produce.[2]

Although some skeptics claim that the levels of pesticide residue remaining on conventional produce are far lower than levels required by the EPA, research shows even these low levels of exposure can cause permanent damage to the developing brain. For example, one review evaluated data from twenty-seven studies and found positive evidence that children and adolescents exposed to organophosphate pesticides (even in utero) exhibited neurodevelopment deficits in intelligence, problem solving, brain processing speed, working memory, fine and gross motor skills, and communication. Further, they had an increased risk of attention and hyperactivity diagnoses.[3] Organic farming doesn't allow organophosphate pesticides.

Unlike conventional farming, organic farms use natural, nonsynthetic pesticides, only if absolutely necessary, to eliminate insects or weeds.

While organic produce can have some pesticide residue, reports show residues are ten to one thousand times lower than levels found on conventional produce and are a result of factors over which the organic farmer has no control, such as residues found in soil, water, or packaging.[4]

STAY DOMESTIC

According to studies by Charles Benbrook, pesticide policy expert and researcher, and his colleagues, imported organic produce is more likely to contain residues of higher dietary risk than is domestically grown organic produce, though still within the EPA tolerance level for organic labeling.[5]

Since the American Academy of Pediatrics reviewed the evidence of children's exposure to pesticides, they now recommend parents reduce or eliminate exposure of pesticides by consuming organic produce, and using organic or integrated pest management practices in and around the home or settings where children spend time.[6] Reducing your family's exposure to pesticides and teaching your children the benefits of organic food will lower long-term exposure and develop positive food choice habits that persist into adolescence and adulthood.

DID YOU KNOW?

The label "natural" or "all natural" has no universal definition and is not regulated by the USDA or the FDA. Every manufacturer can use its own definition, so definitions vary widely. Yet, according to consumer survey data, consumers think the "natural" label means the food is grown without pesticides, contains no genetically modified organisms or artificial ingredients, and is processed without chemical processing aids. Like other unverified food labels, the "natural" label is confusing and misleading to consumers. To be sure your food products are free of pesticides and additives, choose only products displaying the USDA organic seal.[7]

THE CHANGE
CHOOSE ORGANIC FOOD, AND GARDEN AND LAWN CARE, AS MUCH AS POSSIBLE.

PATH TO CHANGE Use the following strategies to reduce your family's exposure to toxic pesticides found in conventional food, gardening, and lawn care.

CHECK THE LABEL All organic products bearing the USDA organic seal must meet USDA strict standards for organics—food must contain at least 95 percent organic ingredients, and the facilities that handle and process the food must be inspected and certified, as well. Alternatively, if a product contains at least 70 percent organic ingredients, it can bear a different label, "Made with Organic Ingredients." Lastly, the PLU (price lookup) or four-digit codes found on stickers of individual pieces of produce can also be used to find organic items. Organic produce has a prefix of "9" before the traditional four-digit PLU code—there are no other prefixes, so you can be sure any produce with a five-digit code starting with "9" is organic.

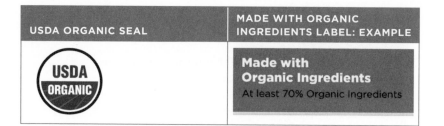

USDA ORGANIC SEAL	MADE WITH ORGANIC INGREDIENTS LABEL: EXAMPLE
USDA ORGANIC	Made with Organic Ingredients At least 70% Organic Ingredients

ASK YOUR LOCAL FARMER Obtaining organic certification costs farmers tens of thousands of dollars, a price tag often out of reach for many small local farms. But choosing to eat locally grown produce often comes with the benefit of personally knowing your local farmer. Ask your farmers which practices they use to manage insects, pests, and weeds.

You may be pleasantly surprised to learn that some local farmers follow organic practices even though they aren't officially certified and are up front about if and when they spray crops.

START WITH THE DIRTY DOZEN   All conventional "pesticide-treated" produce contains residue from chemicals used in farming. The number and amount of pesticides used, however, varies considerably with different types of produce. Each year, the Environmental Working Group (EWG) creates a list of twelve types of produce containing the highest loads of pesticide residue, based on samples analyzed by the USDA. Most varieties included on the Dirty Dozen list have thin, edible skin, such as berries, apples, and pears. To lower your family's pesticide load, buy organic versions of the produce found on the latest Dirty Dozen list, available at www.ewg.org.

SAVE ON CLEAN FIFTEEN   The EWG also creates a Clean Fifteen list of the top fifteen varieties of produce least likely to contain pesticide residues. In many instances, though not all, the varieties of produce found on the Clean Fifteen contain thick skin that is typically peeled before eating, such as avocados, pineapples, onions, cantaloupe, and grapefruit. To save money, purchase conventional varieties of produce found on the latest Clean Fifteen list. Reference www.ewg.org for the most up-to-date list.

WASH AND PEEL NONORGANIC   In conventional farming, pesticides are sprayed on produce and used in fertilizer. Although this won't eliminate pesticide residues entirely, thoroughly washing conventional produce can help reduce your family's exposure.

SHOP AROUND TO SAVE MONEY   There is no doubt organic food costs more than its conventional counterparts, but pricing across grocery chains and online suppliers varies considerably. Save money by comparison shopping for common organic products your family uses. Many low-cost grocers, such as Walmart, Market Basket, Trader Joe's, and Aldi, and membership stores, such as Costco, also offer organic produce at a good price. When your favorite produce is not in season or not available as organic, buy frozen organic versions instead. You can also save money on organic dry goods (such as nuts, seeds, grains, and beans) through online retailers, such as Vitacost or Amazon.

REDUCE EXPOSURE AT HOME   Chronic low-level exposure to pesticides is common in the United States due to the use of insecticides and rodenticides in homes, and the application of herbicides on lawns or in gardens. These products are tracked into your home on shoes and the paws of pets. Children are at higher risk because they are more likely to put unwashed hands in their mouths and to roll around on the floor, increasing their exposure to tracked-in chemicals.[8]

Try organic lawn products   Use composts instead of synthetic fertilizers to make your lawn lush. Compost is an inexpensive natural fertilizer produced from decomposed organic or plant matter. It is rich in nutrients and key to organic farming. Or, use a mulching mower to return clippings to the lawn.

Avoid combination lawn products   Combination products that include pesticides and fertilizers, known as "weed and feed" products, tend to apply higher levels of pesticides than needed.

Weed by hand   Although more strenuous, hand weeding as opposed to applying herbicides can reduce your family's exposure to pesticides. There are many new tools to help make this process easier.

Practice integrated pest management   Also known as "IPM," integrated pest management tries to reduce insecticide use through strategies that naturally deter insects from a specific area. For example, instead of spraying chemicals, reduce the prevalence of rodents and insects by storing food in airtight containers, plugging water leaks, and using bait stations or traps. Additionally, IPM recommends the use of less toxic products when necessary, such as boric acid to deter ants, silverfish, termites, and cockroaches.

LIVE INTENTIONALLY

*The meeting of two eternities, the past and future . . .
is precisely the present moment.*
—HENRY DAVID THOREAU

FOR THOUSANDS OF years, spiritual and religious organizations of all types have taught that mindfulness, or living in the moment, or being present is the most direct path to happiness. According to data analyzed by the founders of TrackYourHappiness.org, our enlightened leaders are right. Data from over five thousand people in eighty countries shows that people are most happy when their minds are not wandering elsewhere, regardless of whether those thoughts are positive or negative.[1]

Successful mindfulness-based programs have been implemented worldwide in a variety of settings and with people of all ages. Studies show that when adults are taught how to live mindfully, using mind-training techniques, breathing exercises, and meditation, they are better able to manage stress and regulate emotions. Further, they have lower blood pressure, enjoy improved immune function, and experience less pain.[2,3,4,5] Children benefit, too. When they are taught mindfulness practices, they are better able to regulate emotions and cope with challenging life situations. They also enjoy greater well-being, experience lower anxiety and depression, and are better able to focus and concentrate.[6,7]

A key component of being mindful is to be deliberate about the choices we make in life, instead of living on autopilot, with people and circumstances around us dictating how our life unfolds. Stepping into the driver's seat of your own life is empowering and helps us feel in control of our personal experiences, regardless of negative situations we may encounter. Living in the moment also requires not being a spectator in your own life, but rather an active participant.

THE CHANGE
PRACTICE LIVING MINDFULLY.

PATH TO CHANGE Live consciously as a family, with intention and purpose, using the following strategies:

TAKE STOCK By understanding how your family's time is spent each day, you can work together to identify opportunities for more purposeful living. For example, according to the Bureau of Labor Statistics, both men and women in households with a child under six years old spend an average of two hours daily watching television.[8] After a long day of work and family chores, television may feel like a much-needed reprieve for parents. However, the collective time spent on television could be used on other interests and passions that bring more joy to life. Use the Time Tracking Assessment in Part III: Tools and Resources to understand how your family spends its time. Track time spent on various activities for both weekdays and weekends. Consider the list of sample activities provided on the worksheet to see which might apply. Then track the minutes spent throughout the day on each activity, rounding to fifteen-minute increments. Finally, add up the total time spent on each activity.

STOP RUMINATION Jon Kabat-Zinn, founder and former executive director of the Center for Mindfulness in Medicine, Health Care, and Society at the University of Massachusetts Medical School, tells us, "Ordinary thoughts course through our mind like a deafening waterfall."

It's important to reflect and process thoughts. However, using excessive amounts of time and energy to analyze everything can impede your family's ability to enjoy the present moment. By carving out dedicated time for reflection through journaling or conversation, you can teach children how to observe their thoughts without overwhelming their life.

PRACTICE MINDFULNESS EXERCISES   Lead your family through mindfulness-based activities and exercises to increase awareness, regulate internal emotions, and become more conscious in life. Practicing together allows you to deepen your relationships and further your learning.

Enjoy singing bowls   Traditional Himalayan singing bowls have been used by Tibetans and monks for centuries in rituals, prayers, meditation, and sound healing. The bowls make a beautiful sound that calms the mind and body. A common way to increase awareness of sound is to have your family members close their eyes and listen closely while one person swirls a wooden mallet to make the bowl sing—once the sound dissipates, have everyone open their eyes again. Repeat.

Breathe   Conscious breathing can benefit your family in many ways: from stopping an impulsive purchase to promoting calm in an otherwise chaotic situation. Use breathing to help you raise awareness of moments throughout the day you might not typically notice. A breathing buddy (such as a stuffed animal) can help inspire and teach young children the power of breath work.

Take a mindful walk   Sarah Rudell Beach, founder of LeftBrainBuddha .com, dedicates a regular family walk as a "noticing" walk, one in which you spend time finding and pointing out to each other things you hadn't noticed in the past. This type of walk teaches children how to literally stop and smell the roses.

Meditate together   Meditation is a powerful practice used to quiet the mind and create space to live in the moment. It is a tool that helps people regulate emotions and connect with their inner self. Children as young as three years old can learn how to meditate—it just may not look the same

CREATE A MIND JAR

IN THE CHILDREN'S book *A Moody Cow Meditates*, by Kerry MacLean, the narrator tells a sweet story about a very moody cow who eventually learns to regulate his emotions using a mind jar.[9] This activity is ideal for children ages three to ten, but it could also be beneficial for parents and teens.

YOU'LL NEED:

+ Pint-sized glass jar with lid
+ Warm water
+ Glycerin (about ¼ cup)
+ Clear liquid hand or dish soap (4 drops)
+ Colorful glitter

DIRECTIONS:

+ Fill the glass jar ¾ full with warm water.
+ Add glycerin to the top ¼ of the jar.
+ Add the drops of soap.
+ Cover the jar tightly and shake until the soap and glycerin are dissolved.
+ Add pinches of glitter, typically 1 tablespoon total, until you've achieved the desired effect.
+ Cover and shake.

Have family members use the mind jar when they are angry, sad, or emotional. Shake it up, and as the glitter settles, imagine emotions dissipating like the glitter in the jar.

as when adults meditate. Refer to Week 12, Just Breathe, for more information about the power of meditation and how to incorporate it into your family life.

LET EMOTIONS COME AND GO Like thoughts, emotions can overtake our minds, preventing us from living consciously. More important, one way children learn how to regulate emotions is by observing how their parents regulate emotions.[10] By practicing mindfulness, parents can learn new tools for regulating their emotions that ultimately benefit their children as well.

SET GOALS In Week 14, Set Goals, we talk about the value of setting goals and intentions and how to help children of all ages become goal setters. Actively setting goals for life encourages your family to live consciously, recognizing that each individual person is responsible for creating the life she desires.

READ BOOKS THAT TEACH MINDFULNESS People of all ages learn through storytelling. Since living consciously is a bit of an elusive concept, stories are a great tool! Look for books that teach children about mindfulness using concepts such as how to pause before reacting, embrace the beauty in life, make conscious choices, find silence, and recognize emotions. Refer to suggestions in the table of Mindfulness-Based Books for Children on the following page.

USE INSPIRING VISUAL CUES Water fountains, rock gardens, and statues of the sitting Buddha are peaceful displays that can promote a sense of calm and act as visual reminders to be present. A simple framed phrase, an illustration, or a piece of jewelry containing the words "Be Here Now" or "Live in the Moment" can also remind family to pause and reset with a focus on the current moment. Encourage each family member to find a personal item that's a reminder to embrace mindfulness.

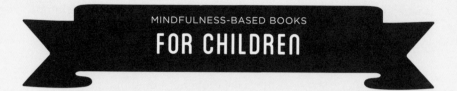

FOR CHILDREN

THOUGH NOT EXHAUSTIVE, the following short list of book recommendations can be used to introduce the concepts of mindfulness to your children.

AGE RANGE	STORIES	WORKBOOKS/GUIDES
2 to 6 years	*Buddha at Bedtime*, by Dharmachari Nagaraja *Anh's Anger*, by Gail Silver *Moody Cow Meditates*, by Kerry MacLean *The Lemonade Hurricane*, by Licia Morelli *What Does It Mean to Be Present*, by Rana DiOrio	*Sitting Like a Frog*, by Eline Snel (for parents)
7 to 12 years	*A Pebble for Your Pocket*, by Thich Nhat Hanh *Milton's Secret: An Adventure of Discovery through Then, When, and the Power of Now*, by Eckhart Tolle *Visiting Feelings*, by Lauren Rubenstein	*The Seven Spiritual Laws for Parents*, by Deepak Chopra (for parents)
13 to 18 years	*Buddha in Your Backpack*, by Franz Metcalf *Dharma Punx*, by Noah Levine	*Fire in the Heart: A Spiritual Guide for Teens*, by Deepak Chopra *The Mindful Teen: Powerful Skills to Help You Handle Stress One Moment at a Time*, by Dzung X. Vo *Wide Awake: A Buddhist Guide for Teens*, by Diana Winston *The Stress Reduction Workbook for Teens: Mindfulness Skills to Help You Deal with Stress*, by Gina Biegel

TAKE CHARGE OF YOUR HEALTH

Health is like money; we never have a true idea
of its value until we lose it.
—Josh Billings

A COMMON CRITICISM OF America's healthcare system is that it's highly effective for disease management but not set up to promote health. Fortunately, the same habits that kept us healthy since the dawn of time still work today—eat fruits and vegetables, exercise daily, sleep eight hours a night, avoid smoking, take your vitamins, get an annual physical exam, follow doctor's orders, and indulge a little. The CDC estimates that by adhering to these habits, 30 percent of heart disease–related deaths, 15 percent of cancer-related deaths, and 28 percent of stroke-related deaths could be prevented each year.[1]

When we skip these health habits, our health can suffer, and we must turn to the healthcare system for support. Before the Internet, when patients received a medical diagnosis and treatment plan from a doctor, it was extremely difficult to explore other courses of action beyond getting a second opinion. Now, health information is readily available at our fingertips: everything from alternative treatment options to the latest scientific research.

According to the Pew Research Center, 72 percent of adults search online for information about health issues, especially diseases and treatment options.[2] Families can use this information to become proactive about their health, achieve better health outcomes, and take ownership of medical decisions for themselves and their families, instead of relying on conventional healthcare to make decisions for us.

When patients participate in their health and medical decisions, it leads to treatment plans that are more consistent with personal values and, per growing research, results in the same or better outcomes for patients.[3,4] For example, a Cochrane review (the gold standard of medical research) found that when patients participated in decision making on whether to take a prescription drug for upper respiratory infections (a treatment approach typically not supported by medical research), antibiotics were prescribed 40 percent less than usual.[5]

There is still a tendency for doctors to make decisions about your health without input from you. Fortunately, a new standard of practice—informing and involving patients in medical decisions—is slowly gaining momentum. Learning how to stay healthy and happy with preventative habits starts at home, particularly since healthy habits developed as a child persist into adulthood. In the same vein, parents can effectively model how to advocate for their own health and wellness.

THE CHANGE
ADOPT PREVENTATIVE HABITS AND TAKE RESPONSIBILITY FOR YOUR HEALTH.

PATH TO CHANGE   Knowledge is power when it comes to your family's health. Teach and model to family members how to be in the driver's seat of their own health and wellness decisions with the following tips:

GET A PRIMARY CARE PHYSICIAN (PCP)   Most insurance plans require that you have a primary care physician. PCPs are instrumental in helping you find required specialists that can further tend to you if health issues should arise. Ask friends or family members for referrals.

OPT IN TO PREVENTATIVE TESTS AND SCREENINGS   Routine tests and screenings provide data vital to maintaining good health.

Blood pressure High blood pressure can lead to heart disease or be a precursor to stroke or kidney disease. Get blood pressure tested annually at the doctor's office or a pharmacy with a blood pressure machine. A healthy, normal blood pressure is around 120/80 in adults.

Cholesterol/blood lipids Blood lipid screening measures LDL, HDL, and triglyceride values. High LDL cholesterol and/or high triglycerides are linked to heart disease. The AHA recommends that adults over age twenty without risk factors have cholesterol checked every four to six years, more if risk factors are present, such as smoking, being overweight, or having high blood pressure or diabetes, or a family history of high cholesterol. The APA recommends that children with a family history of heart attacks or clogged arteries (atherosclerosis), high cholesterol, or an unknown family background should be screened between ages two and ten. Otherwise, children should be screened once between ages nine and eleven and once between ages seventeen and twenty-one.

Blood glucose/diabetes/prediabetes Over seventy-seven million Americans are unaware they have prediabetes, a condition marked by blood glucose levels that are higher than normal but not high enough to be diagnosed as diabetes. People with prediabetes have a much higher risk of developing diabetes—one study estimates 37 percent of individuals with prediabetes will develop type 2 diabetes within four years, if the condition goes unaddressed.[6] The ADA recommends screening every three years for those overweight or over the age of forty-five, when risk of developing diabetes increases. If there's a family history of high blood sugar or other risk factors are present, such as smoking, more frequent screenings are recommended.

Vitamin D Since low vitamin D is associated with a range of conditions, such as type 2 diabetes, multiple sclerosis, and eczema, it is suggested you have your 25-hydroxyvitamin D serum level checked for sufficiency.

Colon cancer As we age, we are more prone to getting colon cancer, the second most common potentially fatal cancer. It's recommended you begin screenings at the age of fifty, earlier if you have family history of colon, intestinal, breast, ovarian, or uterine cancer.

Hearing Though many are reluctant to admit they have hearing loss, it's very common, especially in adults over the age of fifty. If you or any family members strain to hear conversations, require the volume of the TV or radio to be so high that others complain, or need to regularly ask people to repeat themselves, you may have hearing loss. Talk to your family doctor about getting a hearing test.

Osteoporosis screening Women who are postmenopausal with a history of fractures or a family history of osteoporosis should have a bone density test (ideally, a DEXA scan).

Skin cancer As this is the most common type of cancer, and one of the most commonly cured, yearly screenings for skin cancer are highly recommended. Early detection and treatment are vital to curing skin cancer. If a family member has a lot of moles or freckles or previous sunburns or there is a family history of skin cancer, it pays to start screenings at an early age.

Eye doctor All family members should have their vision checked, starting at age three, to identify any vision problems. Even if you have never had vision problems, start getting regular checkups at age forty-five. Glaucoma, a disease that can lead to possible vision loss, becomes more common after forty-five. Early treatment, however, can prevent or delay the onset of serious issues.

Dental Routine dental examinations can reveal many conditions, from vitamin deficiencies to undiagnosed diabetes. It's best for all ages to get a checkup and cleaning twice a year. Between visits, make sure every family member brushes at least twice a day (preferably after meals) using a toothbrush with soft bristles to avoid gum recession, flosses daily (preferably at night), does not smoke or chew tobacco products, and avoids eating sugary foods.

Gynecological exams for women Woman who are eighteen or are sexually active, whichever comes first, should start getting Pap smears. Pap smears help detect reproductive issues, such as human papillomavirus (HPV) and cervical cancer. Early detection makes it easier to treat these conditions. A Pap smear should be conducted at least every three years for women between the ages of twenty-one and sixty-five. For those with a history of abnormal Pap smears, genital warts, sexually transmitted disease (STDs), or multiple sex partners, the doctor may want to conduct Pap smears more often.

Breast cancer screening for women As women get older, their risk of breast cancer increases. Most breast cancers are found in women over the age of fifty. Early detection of breast cancer can make a tremendous difference in effectively treating or curing the disease. Monthly self-exams and yearly breast exams by a doctor are sufficient until the age of forty, at which point a woman should get mammograms every one to two years. If there's a family history of breast cancer, the doctor may suggest getting mammograms earlier and more frequently.

Prostate cancer screening for men Men over fifty should be tested for prostate cancer. African American men or men with a family history of prostate cancer should speak to their doctor to see if it might be prudent to have testing done earlier.

Know what your numbers mean As part of an annual physical exam, your doctor may order routine laboratory tests to screen for anemia, assess your immune system, and evaluate specific cardiovascular markers. Even when a doctor reports your blood tests are normal, understand where your numbers fall within the range for key measures, such as blood pressure or triglycerides. Armed with this information, you can make better choices that may prevent future disease.

ASK MORE QUESTIONS   When a medical decision is needed, research finds that doctors typically provide more information on the positive benefits associated with their recommended treatment options rather than a balanced view of all positive and negative considerations. Ask your practitioner questions about medications, therapies, diagnoses, and alternative treatment options. Insurance reimbursements limit the time doctors can spend with patients, but many doctors are now using email to answer extensive questions. Talk with your physician's office about how to receive answers to your questions.

READ THE FINE PRINT   Since 1994, the number of adults aged forty-five to sixty-four who take prescription drugs regularly has increased by 27 percent. Yet pharmacological medications often come with many undesirable side effects—many of which are not discussed when medications are prescribed to patients. For example, 25 percent of adults aged forty-five to sixty-four are on medication to lower cholesterol (statins), yet Harvard cardiologists raise concern about statins due to the increased risk of developing diabetes.[7,8] If a new medication is truly medically necessary, teach your family the importance of reading the fine print before taking the medication, reviewing and discussing the side effects, and determining if there are any nutritional or lifestyle changes you can make to reduce symptoms and support your body.

TRY COMPLEMENTARY MEDICINE   Using complementary medicine to prevent disease, address common conditions, and maintain good health is a great strategy. For example, chiropractic care can improve chronic ear infections, and acupuncture is a proven therapy for managing chronic pain. Without the backing of major drug companies, the research on many complementary therapies—such as chiropractic care, acupuncture, naturopathy, and herbs—may be more limited, but it still exists. You can learn more about complementary medicine treatments for various conditions and symptoms your family faces on the websites of the National Center for Complementary and Integrative Health (www.nccih.nih.gov) and Natural Medicines (www.naturalmedicines.therapeuticresearch.com).

KEEP ON
THE SUNNY SIDE

Write it on your heart that every day
is the best day in the year.
—Ralph Waldo Emerson

MANY OF US know someone who smiles constantly, can turn a bad situation into a good one, and never seems to have her spirit broken, no matter what type of misfortune she encounters. Some people are frustrated by constant optimism like this; others are inspired by it. Regardless of how you feel, the science is clear—looking on the bright side of life is far more beneficial than not doing so! Overall, research finds people with a positive outlook are healthier than pessimistic people, regardless of their diet or lifestyle.

A positive attitude can improve your performance, especially when faced with setbacks. For example, in one study of male soccer players, researchers found that optimistic players had more completed passes than pessimistic players during the game when their team was not winning.[1] People with a positive attitude prove to be more consistent performers, indicating that hopefulness and perseverance go hand in hand.

Research finds seeing the glass as half full is also protective of your well-being and physical health. Having a sunny attitude is linked to lower blood pressure, cortisol (stress hormone), and inflammation, as well as reduced risk of hypertension, cardiovascular disease, and common respiratory infections.[2,3] In fact, numerous studies have shown that optimistic people have lower mortality rates, especially when faced with a life-threatening disease, such as breast cancer, head or neck cancer, and cardiovascular diseases.[4] Of course, optimism cannot necessarily transform a diagnosis, but people who are hopeful are better able to cope with a curable illness because they see their situation as temporary. They are also more motivated to continue treatment, thereby increasing the chance of survival and healing.

Though some people seem to be born with a more positive attitude, optimism is considered a skill that can be strengthened through conscious, consistent practice. What's more, positivity is powerful and contagious—think of how uplifted you feel after spending time with your spirited, optimistic friend. Working together to boost optimism can lead to a healthier, happier life for your family and your broader community.

DID YOU KNOW?

Optimism and pessimism elicit activity in different hemispheres of your brain. Using functional magnetic resonance imaging (fMRI), scientists observe that people who exhibit an optimistic reaction to a proposed situation have more activity in the left hemisphere (LH) of the brain, whereas their pessimistic peers show more activity in the right hemisphere (RH). The LH of the brain mediates our attentiveness to positive aspects of life and is associated with hopefulness.[5]

THE CHANGE
CULTIVATE A POSITIVE OUTLOOK.

PATH TO CHANGE   Optimism is a powerful habit to cultivate. Arm your family with this critical skill using the following strategies:

OBSERVE YOUR MINDSET   Since positivity and negativity can be infectious, your personal mindset certainly can influence the way your family views life. If you are typically more pessimistic, you can start focusing on your own mindset first. As you begin to demonstrate a more positive way of thinking, your family may take notice, or they could subconsciously shift their attitudes in similar ways. Alternatively, if you are generally an optimistic person, help the rest of your family cultivate this mindset by using deliberate language and having an open dialogue about your hopefulness.

LOOK FOR SILVER LININGS   Help your family navigate misfortunes and persevere with an exercise that shifts their mind to see the glass as half full. Use the Find the Silver Lining Worksheet in Part III: Tools and Resources to come up with a list of typical challenges your family faces in life. Then spend time reassessing each situation and documenting a positive outcome that might result from each misfortune, or a positive action that could be taken to solve the challenge. You can post the results on the fridge or a bulletin board so family members can review often and continue to embrace hopefulness.

FAKE IT   The Facial Feedback Response Theory suggests that the act of smiling makes us feel better and can improve our mood, even if we have to force it.[6] Faking an optimistic attitude by smiling, laughing, and forcing yourself to be more positive may be one of the simplest ways to boost your positivity. Strategically place cues and reminders throughout your environment that elicit a smile or a laugh naturally. For example, place photographs of your family acting silly on your desk. Post sticky notes of

USE POSITIVE PSYCHOLOGY

POSITIVE PSYCHOLOGY THERAPISTS believe performing intentional activities to foster positive emotions (and eliminate negative thinking) can lead to improved optimism. Practice the following evidence-based activities to strengthen your optimism muscle:

+ **REMEMBER YOUR VALUES:** First, write a list of things you value. Then choose one value from your list and write a paragraph about its significance in your life. Help younger children by asking questions and documenting their responses so you can read them back at a future date. Refer to Week 21, Discover Your True North, to learn more about values.

+ **PRACTICE KINDNESS:** Deliberately performing kind acts fosters a more positive outlook, among other health benefits. Use the strategies in Week 36, Spread Kindness, to help your family spread kindness.

+ **SET PERSONAL GOALS:** Choosing goals and tracking progress toward those goals improves self-efficacy. Use tips from Week 14, Set Goals, to engage your family in goal setting for a more positive outlook on life.

+ **EXPRESS GRATITUDE:** Take time each day to identify the things for which you are grateful. Better yet, engage your family members in writing and sending letters of gratitude. Use tips from Week 9, Say Thanks, to learn more about gratitude.

+ **HARNESS PERSONAL STRENGTHS:** List your personal strengths and choose one to use in a new and different way for a week. This practice can be affirming, thereby increasing self-confidence and encouraging one to feel power over circumstance.

+ **POSITIVE AFFIRMATIONS:** Every day, take note of three good things you experienced that day. Share these positive experiences with your family during a shared meal, or document them in a journal so you can reflect back on positive memories and thoughts.

silly phrases on bathroom mirrors in your home. Set cheerful computer alerts. Include notes of encouragement in your children's lunchboxes.

USE MANTRAS   Mantras are words or phrases that represent an attitude, belief, or feeling that you want to embody. Mantras can be specific, such as "I think I can," or more broad, such as "Happiness is everywhere." In mantra-based meditation, the meditator repeats the mantra over and over as a means to focus the mind and remove distractions. Similarly, you can use mantras to guide your response to setbacks and challenges faced in daily life. Adopt a mantra that younger children can understand and use in a variety of settings. Encourage older children to find or create a personal mantra that elicits a positive feeling and may be relevant to current challenges they may be facing.

CALL OUT PESSIMISM   When you notice that your partner, spouse, or child is acting cynical or hopeless from a challenge or setback, recognize the negativity and gently offer a more positive perspective. Teach your family how to recognize negativity as well, so they can also take part in promoting a positive environment. For families who enjoy playful teasing, play a game of finding the "Negative Nelly" within your family and take turns using jokes, discussion, or smiling to turn him or her into "Positive Polly."

TRY COGNITIVE BEHAVIORAL THERAPY (CBT)   The National Association of Cognitive Behavioral Therapists (NACBT) explains that CBT is a form of psychotherapy based on the idea that our feelings and behaviors are caused by personal thoughts rather than external things, such as people or events. CBT teaches individuals to recognize and shift thought patterns in order to modify a particular pattern of behavior, such as shifting to a more optimistic mindset. You can find a therapist certified in CBT on the NACBT website (www.nacbt.org/find-a-therapist) or call your health insurance provider to find a CBT-trained therapist near you.

COOK IN,
EAT TOGETHER

If you really want to make a friend, go to
someone's house and eat with him . . . the people
who give you their food give you their heart.

—CESAR CHAVEZ

AS THE WEALTH of a country increases, its citizens spend more on restaurants and eating out.[1] In America, the 1980s marked a decline in the home-cooked meal.[2] By 2015, for the first time in history, Americans spent more money in restaurants and bars than in grocery stores. According to author and researcher Abigail Carroll, "the American dinner has been in a state of decline for several decades now, and people are not eating together as much as they used to."[3,4] Today's parents are feeling more constrained for time, with more mothers working outside the home, changing family structures, and more hours spent at the office and transporting children to sports and activities. Unfortunately, these downward trends in home cooking and family meals are proving harmful to our health.

Food prepared by restaurants, grocery stores, and fast-food establishments is less nutritious; higher in unhealthy fats, refined carbohydrates, and sodium; and usually doesn't contain organic produce or high-quality meats. When you prepare meals at home, however, you have control over the ingredients used. For instance, you may use healthful oils to sauté foods and dress salads, while most restaurants cook with cheaper, unhealthy vegetable oils (read Week 39, Enjoy Healthy Fats, to learn about the nutritional differences among cooking oils). In one study, individuals who reported cooking and eating at home six to seven nights each week ate a healthier diet containing more fiber, fewer carbohydrates, and less sugar and sodium, even when they weren't trying to lose weight.[5] What's more, the majority of children's meals served at restaurants don't meet nutrition recommendations. According to an analysis by the Center for Science in the Public Interest, only 3 percent of 3,494 children's meal combinations offered by the fifty largest chain restaurants met nutrition standards for children.[6]

Cooking is a beneficial skill regardless of the age at which it's learned. Many studies show adults and children who participate in cooking or food preparation programs not only improve their cooking skills and confidence in the kitchen but also make healthier food choices.[7,8,9] In one literature review, researchers reported that children who participated in cooking classes tended to eat more fruit, vegetables, and dietary fiber; were more willing to try new foods; and had increased confidence in food preparation and choice.[10]

Shared meals strengthen relationships and deepen bonds between family members. Creating a ritual of eating meals together ensures that parents remain connected and influential in the lives of their children, especially as they grow into adolescence. Frequent family meals are associated with lower rates of disordered eating, alcohol and substance abuse, violent behavior, and feelings of depression or suicide among youth.[11,12,13] Further, youth who eat with their families more frequently have higher self-esteem and greater success at school.[14]

By cooking at home and gathering the family to share meals, parents are boosting their families' health, teaching children valuable life skills, strengthening bonds, and creating a steadfast source of familial support.

THE CHANGE
EAT DINNER TOGETHER THREE TO FIVE TIMES PER WEEK, AND COOK AT HOME.

PATH TO CHANGE   The effort required to shift from eating out to cooking at home varies with your individual experience, skills, and interest in cooking. Use the following tips to get started:

SET A GOAL FOR SHARED MEALS   The more you eat together, the more likely you'll benefit. In France, 80 percent of meals are shared with others! Of course, every family is unique. Set a realistic goal for how many meals you'd like to enjoy as a family per week. If your children tend to have a lot of activities, be flexible in scheduling and consider their priorities to make your goal realistic.

TAKE A SEAT   Though modern life can make sitting to eat with family seemingly impossible, a little planning and preparation can ensure success. Eating with children, starting at an early age, helps them become competent eaters. Babies and toddlers observe adults to determine whether food is safe to eat. Preschoolers and children of early primary school age mimic how parents build their plate, test new foods, and choose fruits and vegetables. Make it a priority to sit and enjoy your meal too!

ELIMINATE EXPECTATIONS   Going into family meals with expectations for an experience like those you enjoyed before having children will only set you up for disappointment. Try to enjoy the chaos, embrace the silly moments, ignore the mess, and allow conversation to naturally unfold.

SHARE AND LISTEN   Family meals create a safe space for children to express feelings, process their day, and deepen familial connections. Listen intently to children, and share parts of your own life with them. For example, have family members share three of their favorite experiences of the day and one of their least favorite. Find ways to make sharing and listening fun and routine, especially for young children.

HOME COOKING

TIME-SAVING TIPS:

+ Plan for multiple meals.

+ Chop and store vegetables in advance.

+ Buy prechopped vegetables (when in a bind).

+ Wash and scrub instead of peeling vegetables with edible skins.

+ Cook in batches.

+ Use the main protein in multiple meals.

+ Clean as you go.

+ Invest in a food processor.

+ Mix with an immersion blender.

+ Use a slow cooker to make meals while you're away at work.

+ Roast everything together on a sheet pan.

+ Try a pressure cooker for rapid cooking of rice, beans, and even meat!

SIMPLE TOOLS:

+ Quality chef's knife

+ Wood or bamboo cutting board

+ Vegetable peeler

+ Metal measuring spoons

+ Glass liquid measuring cups

+ Metal or plastic dry measuring cups

+ Large stainless steel or glass bowl

+ Large glass roasting pan

+ Sheet pan/cookie sheet with sides

+ Stainless steel or ceramic large sauté pan

+ Stainless steel large pot with tight-fitting lid

GET COOKING   With a few kitchen tools, a basic recipe, and fresh ingredients, you can create a delicious meal. If you're a novice in the kitchen, start slowly and focus on simple meals. For more experienced cooks, share your love of cooking with family members to create more opportunities for connecting and spending quality time together. Check the tips under Time-Savers for Home Cooking on the previous page to make it a bit less time intensive. And try to get the whole family involved!

Make food they enjoy   Make healthy dishes your family already enjoys to increase confidence in the kitchen. There are numerous ways you can modify a simple meal to avoid boredom. Try using different vegetables (like baked butternut squash fries instead of baked sweet potato fries) and serving foods in various formats. For example, pulled pork or chicken can be served in lettuce wraps, atop simple homemade slaw, or in taco shells.

Use recipes   When getting started, master simple recipes first by making them a couple of times. With experience, you'll have more success when making modifications to suit your family's tastes, such as altering herbs and spices, using different vegetables, or adding toppings. Choose highly rated recipes from popular culinary websites, such as Food Network (www.foodnetwork.com) and Kitchn (www.kitchn.com), or in cookbooks.

Learn the skills   Expand your skill set by taking knife skills classes and cooking classes offered at a nearby adult education center, community college, restaurant, or farm. Alternatively, you can watch videos on YouTube or take classes offered online.

MAKE A WEEKLY PLAN   Determine what you'll eat in advance so you can enjoy time together rather than be overwhelmed by food preparation. Incorporate children into meal planning once they understand what goes into creating a balanced meal (ages eight and up). Consider the tastes of all family members, and include at least one meal component each person can enjoy (Read Week 7, Foster a Positive Relationship to Food, to learn more about helping children develop into competent eaters). Use the Seven-Day and Five-Day Menu Plan Worksheets in Part III: Tools and Resources to plan a week or workweek of meals.

KITCHEN TASKS BY AGE

AGE	COOKING/PREP TASKS	CLEANING TASKS
2 to 3 years	Wash and dry produce. Use a salad spinner. Mash potatoes and other vegetables. Scoop squash from skins. Whisk. Brush vegetables with oil. Add measured ingredients. Stir (in an oversized bowl).	Set napkins on the table. Put silverware at table settings. Put used silverware in the dishwasher.
4 to 6 years	Peel vegetables. Chop produce with kid-sized chef's knife. Form cookies and patties. Roll dough. Measure ingredients. Crack eggs. Start and stop the blender or food processor. Whisk and stir.	Set the table. Rinse lightweight dishes. Put dishes in the dishwasher.
7 to 9 years	Use a real paring or chef's knife. Pound meat. Skewer food. Scoop batter into muffin cups. Open cans with a hand can opener. Scoop processed food out of the food processor.	Put away leftovers. Load and unload the dishwasher.
10 to 12 years and up	Sauté. Use baking pans in the oven. Prepare simple meals by following a recipe.	Provide oversight as needed (such as when cleaning sharp objects).

HAVE STRENGTH IN YOURSELF

What lies behind us and what lies before us are tiny matters compared to what lies within us.

—RALPH WALDO EMERSON

HEALTHY SELF-ESTEEM IS one of the most crucial attributes your family can cultivate for greater happiness, well-being, and success. Positive self-esteem is considered a protective factor against stress and mental illness, such as depression. It is also associated with better survival rates and coping abilities in people who are chronically ill or facing serious medical diagnoses, such as cancer and heart disease.[1] And children with positive self-esteem have higher academic success and stronger reading ability, and eventually become adults who experience greater job satisfaction.

For children, self-esteem develops at a young age and typically remains strong until adolescence. Adolescence is a time when tweens and teens are faced with many life-altering experiences, which can affect their own perceptions of themselves.

YOUR INFLUENCE AS A PARENT

A parent's role in the development of a child's self-esteem is vital and cannot be overestimated. Children are more likely to have strong self-esteem when they have parents who provide warmth and unconditional support. Yet when parents overvalue them and make them feel they are superior to others, children are more likely to exhibit narcissism, even beyond the younger years, a time during which self-absorption is considered developmentally normal.[2] On the other hand, if parents are hypercritical of their child, the child's self-perception can become skewed and low self-esteem may result.

Our life experiences at home, school, and work, and among peers influence and shape our feelings and perceptions of ourselves. For example, if a child is teased at school and also doesn't receive approval, love, and unconditional support from parents and other peer groups, her self-love may take a beating. Additionally, teens and adults who constantly evaluate and compare themselves to celebrities or peers tend to have low self-worth. And, believe it or not, becoming a parent can take a toll on self-esteem, too. In a large study of almost eighty-five thousand women, researchers found that a woman's self-esteem typically declines within the first three years after having a child.[3]

Working as a family to build and strengthen self-worth and self-love increases the likelihood that each of you will flourish and thrive through the ups and downs of life.

THE CHANGE
ADOPT STRATEGIES TO STRENGTHEN SELF-ESTEEM.

PATH TO CHANGE   A healthy self-esteem serves as a solid foundation for health, happiness, and success. Guide yourself and your family in developing a strong sense of self by using the following strategies:

TACKLE EMOTIONS ASSOCIATED WITH SELF-DOUBT   Research finds that when a person experiences emotional distress, it tends to trigger the individual to begin underestimating her abilities. And self-doubt exhibited in childhood can grow over time if left unaddressed. If you notice that you or your child exhibits signs of insecurity and uncertainty, work to identify and acknowledge the emotions or memories that may be the cause of self-doubt.

APPRECIATE UNIQUENESS   Every one of us is unique, and this should be celebrated. Raise consciousness about the importance of being unique by exploring and discovering the unique attributes, skills, and interests of each family member. When a family member starts to feel negative about herself, you can remind her of the qualities that make her unique and engage the entire family in a celebration of her uniqueness.

GIVE EVERYONE A VOICE   With the rumblings against child-centric parenting, you might be inclined to limit input from your child in familial decisions. Before shutting your children out of decisions, however, consider how it feels when you are given a say in important decisions at work or at home. You likely feel respected, flattered, and have more self-confidence. Children begin to build their self-efficacy and inner strength when they have a voice in their own lives. By our giving them a voice, they also learn how to make decisions and live with the consequences of their choices. For example, you can let young children decide which extracurricular activities to join, the books to read each night, the clothes they wear each day, and what to do during family time. Continue expanding the decisions your children are involved with as they grow and mature.

HAVE HEALTHY DISAGREEMENTS   It sounds like a dream to have a tween or teen who follows the rules without discussion. But experts say it is normal for older children—even those who feel adequately supported and loved at home—to begin challenging familial rules in search of more autonomy. Developing independence is a critical developmental milestone for teens. Instead of shutting down disagreement, engage your tween or teen in a respectful argument that gives him the opportunity to advocate for himself and learn how to make independent decisions despite pressure from others, such as you (or his peers). Even if you do not plan to change your rules, you can model for a teen how to have a respectful disagreement by listening to his viewpoint, showing empathy, acknowledging his emotions, staying calm even if he is not, and, if he begins acting disrespectfully, gently reminding him to talk to you with kindness.

DID YOU KNOW?

Preteens who struggle to establish autonomy within their family are also more likely to struggle with being autonomous among friends and peers. One study found that adolescents who were more confident to engage in a disagreement with their mothers at age thirteen were also less likely to use drugs or alcohol, even when peers were using these substances. Researchers find that healthy development of autonomy at home, along with parental support, can protect teens from engaging in deviant behaviors due to peer pressure.[4]

TAKE HEALTHY RISKS   When we do things that challenge us, when we push ourselves to do something a tad uncomfortable, we feel a greater sense of vitality and happiness. And the more we push ourselves outside the boundaries of our comfort zone, the more confident we feel about our abilities. Healthy risk taking boosts self-efficacy and self-confidence. Learn new ways to challenge yourself and your family using tips in Week 34, Push the Boundaries.

KNOW YOUR VALUES   The more an individual knows her values and understands what is truly important to her, the less likely she will feel self-doubt or make choices incongruent with who she is as a person. Our values ground us and guide us when making decisions throughout life. Review Week 21, Discover Your True North, for tips on understanding and celebrating the values of your family.

ESCAPE EXCESSIVE CRITICISM   When another person provides constructive feedback in a positive manner, we are able to internalize the information and use it to improve ourselves. On the other hand, when we receive a constant barrage of feedback, it can hurt our self-esteem; this is especially true for young children. When delivering feedback to loved ones, attempt to deliver it in a warm and friendly manner, instead of being matter-of-fact and overly direct. Avoid too much exposure to any individuals who could be hurting any family member's self-esteem with excessively critical feedback.

COUNTER NEGATIVE SELF-TALK   Self-talk refers to the internal conversations and discussions we have with ourselves. A simple strategy to boost self-esteem is to repeat positive affirmations about yourself aloud. Researchers find making positive statements about oneself improves self-esteem by nurturing and affirming positive versus negative beliefs. Use the Reframe Negative Self-Talk Worksheet in Part III: Tools and Resources to list all the negative thoughts felt by you or a loved one. Next to each thought, write down a counter thought that is positive and uplifting. Another recommended strategy has you write down negative thoughts, then physically crumple up the paper and throw it in the trash as you would another material object. In a series of studies, teens who had physically thrown away their negative thoughts were less likely to be impacted by them later, whereas the teens who had written their thoughts down but not disposed of them had continued to rely on the negative thoughts in their attitudes and actions.[5]

PRAISE CONSCIOUSLY Experts suggest that the nature of the praise we offer to children can significantly influence what the child grows up to value in herself and how she views herself in relation to others. For example, little girls who are constantly complimented on their appearance grow up into adolescents who find it challenging to appreciate and nurture their other positive qualities. Spend more time noticing and praising hard work and effort rather than complimenting appearance or other inborn qualities, such as natural talent for music or athletics.

AVOID ACTIVITIES THAT ENCOURAGE COMPARISONS When we constantly compare ourselves to others, we slowly eat away at our self-worth. Some activities lend themselves to comparison making more than others. For instance, reading tabloids or magazines with airbrushed photos, gossiping, watching reality television shows, and frequently scrolling on social media sites keep us in a superficial, comparing mindset. Reduce these activities within your family; focus instead on activities that are meaningful and highlight the positive qualities of others.

CULTIVATE EMOTIONAL INTELLIGENCE

♡

No one cares how much you know,
until they know how much you care.
—THEODORE ROOSEVELT

EMOTIONAL INTELLIGENCE IS "the ability to monitor one's own and others' feelings and emotions, to discriminate among them and to use this information to guide one's own thinking and actions."[1] People with more emotional intelligence or a higher "EQ" are generally happier and in better health, both mentally and physically.[2,3]

Adults who exhibit higher levels of EQ are better able to work in teams, perform under pressure, manage through job stress, and build a mutually supportive, trusting network of influential relationships within an organization.[4,5] Emotionally intelligent adults also achieve higher performance at work, receive more promotions, are given higher raises, and are rated more positively by their peers and supervisors.[6] In one study, teachers with higher EQ had less job-related stress and burnout—a common reason why teachers change careers within the first five years on the job.[7]

Building EQ takes time and starts in childhood. As parents, we want our children to feel and express their emotions but not be overwhelmed by them. When children are young and just learning to regulate their emotions and feelings, some outbursts and tantrums are par for the course. Once children reach school age, however, those who have not learned to regulate their emotions will face more difficulty in academics, relationships, and life. Yet children who develop higher EQ are able to pay better attention in school, achieve higher academic success, and be more productive in the classroom.[8] Further, children with strong EQ tend to be more caring and empathetic, and therefore better at resolving conflicts with others.[9,10] Emotional intelligence is also associated with reduced risk of unhealthy behaviors in young adults and teens. One study of college students found young men with low EQ were more likely to use alcohol or illicit drugs, exhibit defiant behavior, such as fighting, and have poorer relationships with peers.[11]

YOUR INFLUENCE AS A PARENT

Parents have a fundamental role in helping their children develop emotional intelligence—a role that requires patience, compassion, and fortitude. As we all know, staying calm and offering helpful support when a child has a tantrum is one of the most difficult parts of parenting. It is during these emotionally charged moments we become aware of our own ability to regulate and manage our emotions. Fortunately, experts find that adults can improve their emotional intelligence with concerted effort, benefiting all relationships.[12] For example, one study found that in marriages where at least one spouse exhibited high levels of EQ, both partners reported more satisfaction with the marriage and more positivity about the relationship.[13] And emotional intelligence tends to increase with age and maturity.

DID YOU KNOW?

Teens who have emotional outbursts are not necessarily reverting back to toddler behavior intentionally. According to Deborah Yurgelun-Todd, a neuroscientist and researcher, the teenage brain processes external emotional information differently than the adult brain does. Magnetic resonance imaging (MRI) shows that when faced with an emotionally charged situation, teenagers use a part of their brain that manages emotions, whereas adults use the part of the brain that manages executive controls (more rational thinking). As a result, teenagers who face these situations may respond with a gut reaction or impulsive response that looks more like an outburst than a thoughtful, mature response.[14]

THE CHANGE
CULTIVATE AND DEVELOP
EMOTIONAL INTELLIGENCE.

PATH TO CHANGE Working as a family to build or strengthen emotional intelligence deepens our relationships, can improve performance at work and school, and helps us navigate life's challenges and disappointments. Use the following strategies to deepen the EQ of your family:

ACKNOWLEDGE EMOTIONS Dr. Laura Markham, clinical psychologist, author, and founder of AHA! Parenting (www.ahaparenting.com), explains that children feel heard and see their emotions as valid when parents acknowledge emotions instead of redirecting or dismissing them. Once children feel validated, they eventually become less insistent in their emotional demands and their emotions feel less urgent when they arise. One study showed when parents were more emotionally available and sensitive to their infants, those infants developed into toddlers with more self-control and situational compliance.[15] This philosophy extends to adults as well: one of the most effective ways to develop intimacy with your partner is to validate or acknowledge his feelings, showing you care and value your relationship.

DISCUSS AND EXPRESS EMOTIONS   Talking about emotions with your family teaches children it is acceptable to have feelings. It also gives them the opportunity to identify their feelings and find ways to overcome them with guidance. In one study, two groups of preschoolers were shown illustrated stories. One group then enjoyed free play, while the other had guided conversation about the nature, causes, and regulation of emotions represented in the stories. After six weeks, the children in the conversation group displayed significantly greater gains in emotional comprehension and prosocial behavior (such as helping, comforting, and making peace with others) than did the students who played. What's more, these outcomes remained stable for at least four months, according to follow-up evaluations.[16] If you grew up in a home where feelings were not acknowledged or expressed, it can be particularly uncomfortable and difficult to share feelings. Start by encouraging children to share their feelings, and don't hesitate to seek professional support to help you in this process.

LABEL EMOTIONS   Cultivating a larger vocabulary for describing emotions enables us to accurately express our feelings. Experts explain that once we can pinpoint our true emotions, it is much easier to determine the cause of our emotions and an appropriate regulation strategy. The Mood Meter, a tool designed by the Yale Center for Emotional Intelligence to help toddlers and preschoolers learn to recognize, label, express, and regulate feelings, is available for iOS and Android devices (download at http://moodmeterapp.com/).[17] Researchers have found that regularly using this tool will naturally increase empathy and foster a safe environment for sharing emotions.

SET FAIR LIMITS   Parents who set fair and necessary limits for children are providing opportunities to learn self-control and self-discipline—important skills for everything from financial and physical health to having healthy relationships. When we set limits, we should expect children to feel and express emotions. Dr. Laura Markham explains that when we empathize and accept our children's emotions, they'll learn how to express and accept their feelings and move on from them more quickly. Choose limits that keep children safe and align with values such as being kind and respecting others. But be careful not to set unnecessary or extreme limits, which may cause children to resist and feel resentful.

FIND EMOTIONALLY INTELLIGENT ROLE MODELS   Surround your family with people who know how to express emotions in a healthy manner. Consider the influence coaches, teachers, extended family, and friends have on your children. For example, if a coach screams and yells at players when a game is going poorly, children on the team can think this behavior is normal and acceptable. Instead, look for role models who exemplify healthy emotional intelligence.

INCREASE YOUR EQ   No matter your current level of emotional intelligence, taking actions to increase your EQ is a skill worth honing. Research shows children imitate their parents, especially when it comes to emotional regulation and interactions with other people.[18] Build your EQ by signing up for a reputable coaching program such as "Emotion Coaching" by the Gottman Institute (Emotioncoaching.gottman.com)—a program designed to deepen parents' EQ and their ability to cultivate EQ in their children. Alternatively, you can find a neuro-linguistic programming (NLP) coach who has been trained in social and emotional intelligence.[19]

MANAGE INTENSE EMOTIONS WITH
HEALTHY BEHAVIORS

FEELING EMOTION IS normal. When we don't accept our emotions, however, they get pushed down and can erupt in uncontrollable anger or lead to depression. Use the following tools to help your family manage and move past intense feelings in a healthy way:

+ **COUNTING TO TEN:** Counting to ten is a simple and effective strategy that can help people of all ages manage anger or frustration.

+ **DEEP BREATHING:** Similar to counting, deep breathing or exhaling for twice as long as you inhale calms the body and allows you to release strong emotions.

+ **SELF-TALK:** Offering yourself private words of encouragement and comfort can help instill confidence and resilience when faced with hardships.

+ **REFRAMING NEGATIVITY:** Negative talk can be discouraging and propel us into a downward spiral of negativity. Stop negative thinking and cynical self-talk by reflecting on more positive aspects of a situation.

+ **PHYSICAL DISTANCE OR EXERTION:** Taking time away from an emotionally charged situation allows you to collect your thoughts and release intense emotions without physically or emotionally hurting another person.

+ **SOCIAL SUPPORT:** Shift your current state of emotion by reaching out to friends and family who can listen, give you a hug, or make you laugh during a stressful or upsetting moment.

+ **MEDITATION:** Adopting a regular meditation practice nurtures your parasympathetic nervous system, keeping you more calm—a preventative measure for managing intense emotions.

UPGRADE YOUR MEDICINE CABINET

Leave your drugs in the chemist's pot if you can heal the patient with food.

—HIPPOCRATES

WHEN ONE PERSON in the family gets sick with a cold, the flu, or a stomach bug, it takes a toll on the entire family. From unexpected days out of work to missed school assignments, the added stress from illness sends parents searching desperately for doctors and urgent care clinics to prescribe medications that speed up the healing process. Yet research indicates we might be looking for relief in the wrong place.

According to the Centers for Disease Control (CDC), one in three prescribed antibiotics is unnecessary. And more than half the antibiotics prescribed to treat sinus infections, middle ear infections, bronchitis, pneumonia, flu, and allergies are unnecessary because the majority of these infections are viral and do not respond to antibiotics.[1] Similarly, most gastrointestinal infections are self-limiting and will resolve on their own.[2]

Further, when it comes to symptom relief, many over-the-counter medications (OTC) we turn to may not be as safe as we once thought.

Acetaminophen (the active pain relief ingredient in Tylenol and other cold and flu medicines), for example, produces a byproduct that is highly toxic to your liver when metabolized. According to Professor Gary Peltz, M.D., Ph.D., "Severe liver damage can occur in as little as two or three times the recommended dosage of acetaminophen...a real problem to consider given so many pediatric OTC medicines contain acetaminophen."[3]

TOXICITY AND OVERDOSE

According to the CDC, over seventy thousand children visit emergency rooms each year for accidental overdoses on OTC drugs: 9.3 percent for acetaminophen, 7.3 percent for cough and cold medications, and 5.3 percent for nonsteroidal anti-inflammatory drugs (such as ibuprofen).[4]

We can protect our children from accidental overdose with careful dosing, but many children's medications are also laden with unhealthy artificial colors and flavors and nasty preservatives. Some of these ingredients have been found to cause hyperactivity in children or adverse reactions such as allergies, asthma, and headaches.

Taking control of your family's health starts with prevention through a healthy lifestyle of quality nutrition, physical activity, adequate sleep, and stress management. When faced with an acute illness, however, using effective natural remedies (free of toxic chemicals) can help your family avoid spreading infection and manage icky symptoms.

DID YOU KNOW?

Having a child increases the number of weeks the average family is sick each year from 7 percent (three to four weeks) to 35 percent (eighteen weeks).[5] And if you have a large family, with at least five children, on average you'll be sick for more of the year than not—65 percent (thirty-four weeks) of the year.

THE CHANGE
STOCK YOUR MEDICINE CABINET WITH NUTRIENTS AND NATURAL REMEDIES TO PREVENT ACUTE ILLNESS AND REDUCE DURATION OF SYMPTOMS.

PATH TO CHANGE   Take a preventative approach to prevention by stocking your medicine cabinet with nutrients shown to support good health, as well as natural medicines to support them in times of illness:

ADOPT A PREVENTATIVE MINDSET   While it may seem impossible to avoid illness when you have children, adopting a preventative mindset can reduce both the spread of infection to other family members and the duration and intensity of symptoms. Ensure that your family gets a healthy diet high in fruits and vegetables, regular exercise, fresh air, and adequate hours of high-quality sleep, and manages stress.

SUPPLEMENT   Even people who eat *extremely* healthy diets can be missing adequate amounts of key nutrients. Natural depletion of soil on farms reduces nutrient levels in our food, as does exposure to light, heat, and oxygen.[6] Ensure that your family is getting adequate nutrients by incorporating high-quality, food-based supplements into your daily routine:

<u>Multivitamins</u> Some evidence shows that the human body more effectively processes vitamins derived from food sources than those from synthetic materials. Choose a food-based multivitamin/multimineral supplement containing the full array of nutrients required for good health to ensure that you're getting adequate nutrition. Multivitamins are available in a variety of forms including pills, tablets, powders that can be mixed in water, and naturally sweetened gummies for younger family members.

<u>Vitamin D3</u> Vitamin D is critical to the health of your bones, heart, and brain, as well as your immune system. Some experts suggest 75 percent

ADD TO YOUR MEDICINE CABINET

STOCK YOUR HOME with the following natural remedies to address acute symptoms of common conditions.

REMEDY	USE	DELIVERY
Arnica cream or pellets	Reduce pain associated with muscle tension, bruises, and scrapes	Rub cream onto skin; take pellets orally.
Chamomile tea (organic)	Support healthy sleep	Brew tea and drink.
Coconut water (unsweetened, organic)	Rehydrate the body	Drink.
Echinacea tincture	Shorten duration of cold symptoms	Mix into water or juice, as directed on the label.
Elderberry syrup	Boost immune system to prevent flu; shorten duration of flu symptoms	Take via spoon, as directed on the label.
Garlic	Boost immune system to fight cold and flu symptoms	Crush into hot water to steep for 10 minutes; strain, add honey, and drink.
Garlic mullein ear drops	Reduce earache	Add to ear as directed.
Ginger	Support upset stomach	Crush into hot water to steep for 10 minutes; strain, add honey, and drink.
Magnesium (powder for kids, capsules for adults)	Reduce pain associated with migraine; use magnesium citrate form for constipation	Mix into water and drink.

CONTINUES...

REMEDY	USE	DELIVERY
Manuka honey	Improve healing of cuts and scrapes	Add dollop to cuts and cover.
Probiotic— *Lactobacillus Rhamnosus* GG strain	Shorten duration of acute diarrhea	Mix capsule contents into applesauce or add to juice.
Probiotic— *Saccharomyces boulardii* strain	Prevent antibiotic associated diarrhea; shorten duration of infectious diarrhea	Mix capsule contents into applesauce or add to juice.
Quercetin (chewable for kids)	Improve allergy symptoms	Kids chew; adults take a capsule with water.
Raw honey	Suppress cough; reduce pain associated with sore throat * Note: Do not give to infants under the age of one year.	Take 1 teaspoon, three or four times per day.
Vitamin B6 (adults)	Reduce pain associated with migraines	Take a capsule with water.
Vitamin C (powder)	Boost immune system to prevent colds; shorten duration of cold symptoms	Mix into water. Drink.

or more of the U.S. population could be deficient in vitamin D. Vitamin D is synthesized in the body through a chemical reaction in the skin that results from sun exposure. In the winter in the Northern Hemisphere, however, the sun is not strong enough to allow for vitamin D synthesis. Therefore, a daily supplement is recommended. See Week 6, Befriend the Sun, to learn more about vitamin D supplementation.

Omega-3 Omega-3 fats are critical for heart and brain health; they are also considered essential nutrients because we can get them only from our food. If your family isn't eating three servings of low-mercury, high omega-3 fatty fish weekly, then it is important to supplement daily with omega-3 fish oil. Choose cod liver oil or krill oil for an omega-3 supplement that also naturally contains vitamin D. Fish oil is available in capsules and liquid, often flavored with lemon or strawberry to make the taste more palatable.

Vitamin C Although many animals can synthesize vitamin C, humans cannot due to a genetic mutation in our DNA. Vitamin C, however, plays a critical role as an antioxidant in the body and in the production of collagen. Taking vitamin C daily boosts the immune system and lowers the incidence of cold symptoms. Food-based vitamin C powders are widely available and can be mixed with water, making it easy for children to digest.

SUPPORT THE GUT Over 80 percent of the immune system resides in the digestive tract. Therefore, when the body is digesting and eliminating food effectively, it has more energy and resources to fight off infection. Probiotics are live microorganisms shown to aid digestion, regulate the immune system, produce substances to inhibit bacterial growth, and support the health of the mucosal lining in your gut.[7] You can find probiotics in capsules or powder form that can be mixed in liquid for young children. Most high-quality probiotic products include a broad range of bacterial species and must be refrigerated.

CHOOSE A QUALITY SUPPLEMENT MANUFACTURER Supplements are regulated under the Dietary Supplement Health and Education Act (DSHEA). Unlike pharmaceutical drugs or many OTC medications, dietary supplements are considered to be foods and do not require the same level of rigor of testing, safety, or efficacy. Therefore, it is important to choose supplements produced by high-quality manufacturers. You can work with an integrative nutritionist or M.D. to source supplements, or use Labdoor (www.labdoor.com) to find which brands rank highest on their tests for label accuracy, product purity, nutritional value, ingredient safety, and projected efficacy.

IMPROVE CHILDREN'S OTC MEDICINES Children's OTC medications are flavored and colored to make them more attractive to children. Most brands use synthetic chemicals for dyes and flavoring—additives associated with undesirable reactions, including hyperactivity. Choose brands committed to using dye-free, natural but effective ingredients for children's medications, such as Zarbee's Naturals and Gaia Kids.

TRY HOMEOPATHY Homeopathy was the dominant form of medicine practiced in the United States until the nineteenth century. Homeopathic remedies are available in sucrose-based dissolvable pellets or water-based tinctures and sprays; the medicine they contain is infinitesimally diluted so the final product does not contain any trace of the original medicine.[8] It is because of this that many Western medical doctors view these products as relatively ineffectual. Despite dissent, however, anecdotal evidence and limited scientific evidence shows homeopathic medicines can be beneficial. Visit your local natural foods store or pharmacy to find the right products for your family. Or search on www.homeopathy .org/find-remedy to find the right remedy for your symptoms.

KICK THE COW (NOT LITERALLY)

The calcium theory has probably done more to damage our health than any single theory in the history of humanity.
—DAVID WOLFE

IT'S UNDENIABLE: AMERICA has a love affair with dairy. The average American eats nearly thirty-three pounds of cheese annually—a threefold increase since 1970.[1] Yogurt consumption has gone up a whopping seventeen times in the same time frame. Although dairy in its many forms is delicious, our love of it is proving harmful to our health.

For starters, dairy is loaded with specific types of saturated fatty acids shown to be inflammatory and artery clogging. Second, most yogurts are full of added sugar; excess added sugar is linked to obesity, type 2 diabetes, high triglycerides and low HDL, and heart disease.[2,3] Harvard researchers followed over 190,000 men and women for several decades to understand the relationship between dairy fat and risk of cardiovascular disease. They found that people who replaced calories from dairy fat with fats from vegetables or polyunsaturated fats were 24 percent less likely to develop cardiovascular disease.[4]

Americans can't be faulted for eating too much dairy. The famous "Got milk?" campaign of the 1990s had Americans convinced dairy was essential for strong bones, especially for growing children. Fast-forward two decades, however, and research has proved dairy isn't as effective at maintaining bone health as scientists once thought. The Nurses' Health Study, which followed nearly seventy-three thousand women for over eighteen years, found milk consumption did not produce any protective effect against fractures.[5] Another published review found adding calcium in the form of dairy products did not result in increased bone density of children or young adults.[6,7] Finally, a study that followed over 6,700 girls from ages nine to fifteen showed no correlation between high levels of milk consumption and lower risk of stress fractures.[8]

Despite the latest research findings, the USDA continues to recommend two to three servings of dairy each day, depending on your age. Fortunately, in 2011, experts at Harvard's School of Public Health and Medical School took a stand against the promotion of dairy for good health and removed it from Harvard's Healthy Eating Plate, an alternative to the USDA's MyPlate. Further, conventional medicine is also starting to recognize a documented connection between dairy and other medical conditions, including asthma, chronic bronchitis, chronic ear infections (in children), colic, eczema, and even sinus conditions.

There is other good news: families can boost their bone and heart health and keep their waistlines in check by choosing alternative sources of calcium.

DID YOU KNOW?

Drinking low-fat dairy products may be harmful to your waistline. A longitudinal study that followed nearly thirteen thousand children from ages nine to fourteen found those who consumed skim or 1 percent milk versus full-fat milk had higher weight gain, as measured by body mass index. Lower-fat dairy products are not as satisfying as their full-fat counterparts; therefore children who consume these products tend to eat more calories to compensate.[9]

THE CHANGE
GET CALCIUM FROM NONDAIRY SOURCES.

PATH TO CHANGE   Strengthen bones and improve your family's heart health by choosing nondairy forms of calcium:

CROWD OUT DAIRY   Restricting dairy from your family's diet can backfire, causing family members to eat more dairy outside the home. Use a technique practiced by health coaches and nutritionists worldwide, called "crowding out." Instead of completely restricting dairy, crowd it out with other delicious nondairy foods. For example, if dairy-filled lasagna is a Sunday favorite, switch to a nondairy favorite such as pulled pork tacos.

ENJOY GREENS AND BEANS   Many varieties of beans and dark leafy greens are high in calcium. For example, two cups of cooked collard greens packs in over 500 mg of calcium, and just one cup of beans contains 200 to 300 mg of calcium (compared to 300 mg in a glass of milk). Add beans—such as chickpeas, black, white, pinto, or kidney beans—to tacos, soups, and stews, or puree them into dips. Incorporate greens into everything from egg dishes to smoothies. Refer to the following "Eat Your Greens" box for more ideas.

CHOOSE ALMONDS   Most varieties of nuts contain some calcium, but almonds are by far the most calcium-rich variety. Just ¼ cup of whole almonds provides 95 mg of calcium. Pair almonds with a healthy fruit for a well-balanced afternoon snack. Use almond butter in place of peanut butter on a sandwich, or with celery, apples, or banana slices. Finally, try making healthy homemade baked goods using almond flour for a delicious calcium-rich treat.

GIVE FERMENTED SOY A TRY   Soybeans are very rich in calcium, with 500 mg in 1 cup. High intake of soy, however, raises health concerns, due

EAT YOUR GREENS

BOOST YOUR FAMILY'S intake of greens with these cooking tips:

+ **FRITTATAS AND SCRAMBLES:** Delicate greens, such as spinach and baby kale, add color and texture to egg dishes without sacrificing flavor.

+ **SOUPS:** Use robust greens, such as collard greens and kale, in big hearty soups during winter months. Cut greens into thin ribbons or tear them into small pieces so your family gets a dose in every bite.

+ **SMOOTHIES:** Add at least 1 to 2 cups of leafy greens to your smoothies. If needed, include naturally sweet fruit, such as bananas, oranges, peaches, or mangos, to balance the flavor of the greens.

+ **MEATBALLS, BURGERS, CASSE-ROLES:** Sneak greens into favorite dishes that are already full of robust flavor. You'll see the greens in meatballs but you'll barely taste them.

+ **SALADS:** Prepare salads that pack a more powerful punch of calcium by including high-calcium greens, such as baby kale, spinach, arugula, and cabbage.

+ **JUICE:** Whereas fruit juices are loaded with sugar, green juices are loaded with vitamins, minerals, and phytonutrients. Use a one-quarter of an apple or carrot to make green juice slightly more palatable if needed.

+ **SAUTÉED:** A side dish of sautéed greens, such as bok choy, kale, or Swiss chard, can be a perfect addition to any midweek meal. Make them extra tasty by cutting greens into thin ribbons and adding herbs and spices, such as fresh garlic, ginger, or spicy red pepper.

+ **ROASTED:** Broccoli is a calcium superhero. Make it more flavorful by drizzling broccoli florets with extra-virgin olive oil and 1 tablespoon soy sauce or tamari, and sautéing it with sliced garlic.

to the estrogenic properties of soybeans. Fermented soy products such as miso and tempeh are a better alternative. Buy miso in small containers to easily make homemade miso soup. Serve tempeh in a stir-fry instead of meat slices for a delicious vegetarian protein option.

BLACKSTRAP MOLASSES   Molasses is the liquid byproduct that remains after sugarcane or sugar beets are processed into sugar granules. Unlike sugar, which is void of any nutrients, molasses contains calcium, iron, vitamin B6, selenium, and magnesium. Use molasses instead of other sweeteners in oatmeal or hot whole grain cereal, smoothies, and home-made baked goods.

DON'T SKIMP ON VITAMIN D   To absorb calcium properly, your body needs adequate levels of vitamin D. If your vitamin D levels are low, which is a common issue for many, it will be difficult to absorb calcium from your food, regardless of how much calcium is in your diet. Read Week 6, Befriend the Sun, for tips on getting adequate vitamin D through sun exposure and supplementation.

GET VITAMIN K2   Excess calcium in the blood will calcify or harden your arteries in the same way it strengthens bones. The role of vitamin K2 is to move calcium from your blood to other areas of your body, such as bones and teeth. Nondairy sources of vitamin K2 include liver, grass-fed meat, and egg yolks.

AVOID CALCIUM LOSS   Calcium not absorbed in the intestinal tract is lost through urine. Diets high in sodium, as well as high-protein diets such as paleo and Atkins, can increase calcium loss in urine. Be mindful of your family's sodium and protein intakes to improve calcium absorption while also improving blood pressure. Choose whole foods over processed foods or prepared foods, which are often laden with excess sodium.

GO GLOBAL

Earth is a small town with many neighborhoods
in a very big universe.
—**Ron Garan**

We are living in a rapidly globalizing world where the next generation of children will live, work, and travel globally, more than any previous generation. Research finds that people who have multicultural experiences are more innovative and creative problem solvers and better at conflict management, can adapt in unfamiliar situations, and achieve greater career success.[1,2]

First, learning and understanding a second language improves cognitive abilities, intelligence, memory, and problem-solving abilities, and can ward off age-related cognitive losses.[3] Also, children and teens who speak a second language perform better on standardized tests and experience higher academic achievement.[4] Scientists find that to manage between two languages, bilingual people are constantly exercising parts of the brain responsible for sensory processing and mental control, resulting in more fine-tuned auditory function and more neural networks in the brain.[5]

Better cognitive control is one reason why people with cross-cultural experiences are typically more creative problem solvers, too. For example, a series of studies conducted by researchers from Northwestern

University and INSEAD found that bicultural people, or those who have lived abroad and identify with the cultures of their home country and another country, were more creatively minded and innovative, and also achieved higher rates of promotion and career success.[6] Another study found that people with various types of multicultural experiences possessed a more open attitude toward foreign cultures, were more creatively minded, and were more successful in solving problems.[7]

Now, more than ever before, global and multinational organizations are demanding that college graduates and potential employees have relevant international experience. In a 2014 survey, the National Association of International Educators (NAFSA) discovered that 39 percent of U.S.-based companies missed out on international business opportunities due to the lack of multicultural skills of staff.[8] Despite the demand for these skills, many advocacy organizations, such as the Committee for Economic Development and NAFSA, report that the U.S. education system is not providing American students with adequate global education and training to meet the needs of global companies.

At home, you can prioritize multicultural experiences to ensure that your children (and you) are prepared for opportunities in the future job market. Not only will you enjoy the experiences of broadening your exposure to the rest of the world, but you will also benefit from improvements in cognitive functioning and protection from mental decline.

THE CHANGE
DEEPEN YOUR MULTICULTURAL EXPERIENCES.

PATH TO CHANGE   Raising a family that is open to other cultures and has some multicultural experiences is a lifelong journey. Practice the following strategies to broaden your family's horizons and begin increasing your exposure to the world:

EMBRACE YOUR OWN HERITAGE   Having a deep understanding of your own culture and heritage sparks curiosity and interest in other cultures, too. Find ways to celebrate and commemorate the countries from which your ancestors originated. For example, if you have Native American origins, visit a museum or cultural center dedicated to Native American history; if your ancestors hail from Ireland, engage your family in a spirited celebration of St. Patrick's Day. Start by choosing culturally relevant activities that are fun and entertaining so your children will be inspired and even more curious about their heritage.

PRIORITIZE A SECOND LANGUAGE   For families that are not bilingual, experts suggest children as young as three years old can start learning a second language. You can also support second language learning at home by enrolling your family in a local language program offered through a community college or university. Hire a tutor to support the whole family. Or get started immediately using online language learning programs such as Rosetta Stone, Pimsleur, or Mango Languages (free through public libraries), or the latest language learning apps.

EXPLORE CULTURAL EVENTS   Multicultural festivals and celebrations include food, music, dancing, and goods that represent a specific area of the world or country. Attending these events is an entertaining way to immerse your family in another culture without having to leave the country.

COOK INTERNATIONAL CUISINE   For families who enjoy cooking and eating, expand your cultural mindset by incorporating international dishes into your meal plans. Expand the benefits by bringing the entire family to an international grocery store to shop for ingredients. And while cooking together, listen to music from the country or region associated with the specific dish.

TALK CURRENT EVENTS   Engage your family in age-appropriate discussion about the latest in global current events to broaden their understanding of the injustices in the world and learn how people in other countries live. For younger children, select topics that they can relate to and that won't scare them, such as inequality of education, hunger, and disaster relief. Consider whether older children and teenagers are mature enough to understand heavier topics, such as war and human trafficking.

TRAVEL GLOBALLY   If your budget allows, taking an international vacation provides a fun, unique way to experience another culture. On your trip, dedicate time to visit tourist attractions as well as safe places that are enjoyed by the local people, such as bazaars, restaurants, and national parks. Alternatively, your family can travel abroad without leaving home through participation in global education programs such as Little Passports (www.littlepassports.com) or Cultured Owl (Culturedowl .com). As a member of these subscription-based services, your family will receive a box of educational materials about a different country each month to facilitate global learning.

GLOBALIZE YOUR DÉCOR   A fun way to incorporate a global mindset into your family life is to add global elements to your home's common areas, such as world maps and inspiring photos of international places of interest. Better yet, display photos from international trips that you and your spouse have taken, or from trips taken by close friends or family. Use this décor to promote worldly discussions or as a simple reminder that the world is vast. When talking about current events, cooking international cuisine, or learning about a new country, point out the countries of interest on the maps so children can visualize their world.

BUY FAIR TRADE

Use your purchasing power to help global artisans earn a fair wage. Fair trade gifts are often packaged with little booklets that offer details about the artisans, including where they live and how the fair wage helps them provide for their family. Your investment can also be used to start a dialogue with your family about other cultures and countries. Ten Thousand Villages (www.tenthousandvillages .com) is one of the world's oldest and largest fair trade organizations. Or purchase handmade, stylish jewelry from Noonday Collection (www.noondaycollection.com), a fair trade organization supporting female entrepreneurs locally and abroad.

VOLUNTEER ABROAD   For families with older children, volunteering abroad is a fun, unique, and relatively inexpensive way to immerse yourself in another culture, while also giving back to the community. Many religious organizations plan annual mission trips that bring faith and support to citizens of third world countries. Or you can plan your own trip with Global Volunteers (www.globalvolunteers.org), one of the world's longest-running vacation volunteering providers, or Global Vision International (www.gvi.usa.com), an organization that specializes in youth volunteer travel. Teenagers who go abroad before college are given the opportunity to gain a deeper understanding of the world's problems while experiencing a new culture and connecting with other like-minded teens.

SPONSOR A CHILD   Each year, over 23,000 foreign exchange students attend secondary school in the United States.[9] American families serve as host families, welcoming foreign students into their home and providing housing, food, necessities, and a nurturing environment while the teen attends school. Hosting a foreign student for an entire year is a big commitment, but many families who have hosted rave about the opportunities it provides for teaching diversity and appreciation for different cultures and ways of living. Find a designated sponsor program to join on the State Department's website (https://j1visa.state.gov/participants/how-to-apply/sponsor-search/). If hosting is not possible, consider sponsoring education or training for an underprivileged child who lives in a developing country. This gives you the opportunity to develop a relationship with the sponsored child by writing to each other throughout the year. A reputable organization to consider is Ark of the Rainbow (www.arkoftherainbow.org).

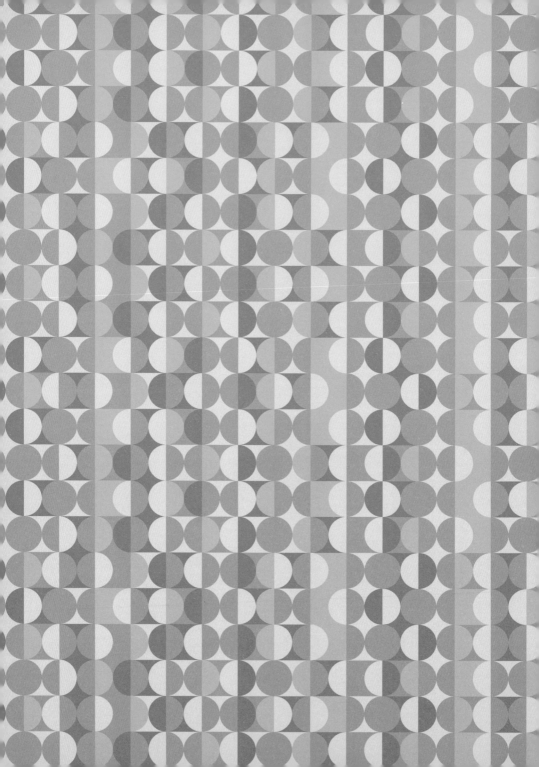

··· PART III ···

TOOLS AND RESOURCES

MEDIA INVENTORY WORKSHEET

Use this template to help each family member log the number of hours each day spent on each of the devices listed. Print out a week's worth of worksheets for each family member. Then, log the number of hours specific to work, school, or personal use in the designated columns. Tally up the hours spent on each device, as well as the total amount of hours spent on all screens per day. Set a goal of how much screen time you'd like to cut out of your week. Write these numbers in the right-hand column, "Goal."

TECHNOLOGY TYPE	HOURS PER DAY		TOTAL	GOAL
	WORK OR SCHOOL RELATED	PERSONAL		
Television/Movie				
Video Games				
Television Screen Total:				
Computer				
Video				
Internet				
Any Software/Application				
Email/IM Chat				
Computer Screen Total:				
Smartphone/Mobile				
Internet				
Text/Messaging				
Video				
GPS Navigation				
Gaming				
eReader App				
Mobile Screen Total:				

TECHNOLOGY TYPE	HOURS PER DAY		TOTAL	GOAL
	WORK OR SCHOOL RELATED	PERSONAL		
Internet				
Text/Messaging				
Video				
Book				
Tablet/eReader Total:				
Cinema				
Other				
Cinema and Other Total:				
MEDIA TOTAL:				

DEEPENING GRATITUDE WORKSHEET

The following questions can be used as prompts to help family members deepen their gratitude for others.[1] Ask these questions after someone has performed an act of kindness for your child, such as giving him a gift or sharing possessions.

ATTACHING VALUE TO HELP OR GIFTS

- When did someone help you or give you a gift that was fun or interesting?

....

....

- Why did the person do this act of kindness or give you the gift?

....

....

COST TO THE BENEFACTOR

- Did they go out of their way for you?

....

....

- What did they give up to do this act for you?

....

....

- Was there a cost to the person (for example, time, money)?

....

....

INTENTION OF THE BENEFACTOR

- Why do you believe they did this for you?

....

....

- How are they investing in you through the help or the gift?

....

....

- What benefits did this person receive from helping you or giving you a gift?

....

....

YOUR REACTION

- How did receiving this help or gift make you feel?

....

....

- What do you think you can do to show your appreciation?

....

....

SMARTER GOALS WORKSHEET

Use SMARTER questions to set your family's goals:

Is it specific?
What do you want to accomplish?

....

....

What steps are necessary to achieve the goal?

....

....

Is it Measurable?
How will you measure the results?

....

....

Is it Actionable?
Do you have the skills to achieve the goal?

....

....

What or who else do you need to accomplish this goal?

....

....

Is it Relevant?
Does this goal match your needs and values?

....

....

Can you accomplish this goal, considering all of your current commitments?

....

....

Is it Time-bound?
When do you want to achieve this goal?

....

....

What can be accomplished in a few days? Weeks? Months?

....

....

Is it Emotionally inspiring?
What is most exciting about achieving this goal?

....

....

How will your life change if you achieve this goal?

....

....

Is this goal Readjustable?
Can you adjust the timing, actions, or activities of this goal, if needed?

....

....

When will you decide whether this goal needs to be readjusted?

....

....

EXPLORE YOUR VALUES WORKSHEET

Use the following questions to help you discover the values you prioritize. After both you and your partner complete the questions individually, share your answers and use the results to determine which values you want to instill in your family. The sample list of values found in Week 21, Discover Your True North, can inspire your exploration.

Which aspects of your life contribute to your happiness?

....

....

What do you like to celebrate and reward?

....

....

How do you define success?

....

....

What do you spend your money on?

....

....

What words would people use to describe you?

....

....

What energizes you? What depletes you?

....

....

NARROW DOWN TO THREE:

Which three values in the list in Week 21 do you cherish most?

....

....

Which of the values do you act on consistently?

....

....

What are you willing to fight for and make sacrifices for?

....

....

SPIRITUAL BELIEFS WORKSHEET

Use the following abbreviated list of questions to explore your spiritual views. Share your answers with your partner or spouse so you can understand each other before sharing with the rest of your family.

What does spirituality mean to you?

Do you consider religion and spirituality to be similar or different? How so?

Do you believe in god, a divine presence, or a higher power? What is it? Where do you find it? How does it fit into your life?

What does spirituality bring to your life?

Is there a moral set of truths or principles that you adhere to?

Why do you think there is evil and suffering in the world?

What do you believe happens after someone dies? Do you believe in heaven?

....

....

How do you connect with your spiritual self?

....

....

How do you fit into the world? What is your purpose?

....

....

How do you want your family to benefit from having a spiritual self?

....

....

SEVEN-DAY WEEKLY MENU PLAN WORKSHEET

Use the following chart as a template for planning your meals each week. Reduce the time it takes to prepare dinner in the middle of the week by chopping vegetables or preparing a sauce in advance—use the last column to keep track of these activities.

	BREAKFAST	LUNCH	DINNER	ADVANCE DINNER PREP
Monday				
Tuesday				
Wednesday				
Thursday				
Friday				
Saturday				
Sunday				

FIVE-DAY WEEKLY
MENU PLAN WORKSHEET

(includes snacks for young children)

Use the following chart as a template for planning your meals and snacks each week. Reduce the time it takes to prepare dinner in the middle of the week by chopping vegetables or preparing a sauce in advance—use the last row to keep track of these activities.

	MONDAY	TUESDAY	WEDNESDAY	THURSDAY	FRIDAY
Breakfast					
Mid-morning snack					
Lunch					
Afternoon snack					
Dinner					
Advance prep					

PANTRY AND FRIDGE SWAP WORKSHEET

Use this worksheet to keep track of the packaged and processed foods for which you would like to find additive-free options. Start by finding healthier alternatives for family favorites; once that is complete, move on to find swaps for the remaining foods.

FOOD TO SWAP	ADDITIVES INCLUDED	ALTERNATIVES TO TRY

KIND ACTS TRACKING WORKSHEET

Use this worksheet as a template for tracking the kindness that each family member shows and receives within the week.

	MY KIND ACTS	KIND ACTS BY OTHERS
Monday		
Tuesday		
Wednesday		
Thursday		
Friday		
Saturday		
Sunday		

How did it feel to be kind to others? Choose five to ten words to describe your emotions.

....

....

How does it feel when another person is kind to you? Choose five to ten words to describe it.

....

....

TIME TRACKING ASSESSMENT

Use the following template for each day of the week to track how each family member spends his or her time and to assess whether the time could be spent on more purposeful activities.

Step #1: Review the list of sample activities. For each day of the week, enter the activity performed for each thirty-minute slot.

Possible activities: work, education, commuting, household activities (cleaning, laundry, food preparation, cooking), shopping for goods or services, personal care for self, sleep, caring for family members, civic/volunteer/religious activities, playing outside, exercise, television, internet surfing, telephone/online chat, leisure, creative activities

DAY OF WEEK: _____

TIME OF DAY	ACTIVITY NAME
5:00–5:30 a.m.	
5:30–6:00 a.m.	
6:00–6:30 a.m.	
6:30–7:00 a.m.	
7:00–7:30 a.m.	
7:30–8:00 a.m.	
8:00–8:30 a.m.	
8:30–9:00 a.m.	
9:00–9:30 a.m.	
9:30–10:00 a.m.	
10:00–10:30 a.m.	
10:30–11:00 a.m.	
11:00–11:30 a.m.	

11:30 a.m.–12:00 p.m.	
12:00–12:30 p.m.	
12:30–1:00 p.m.	
1:00–1:30 p.m.	
1:30–2:00 p.m.	
2:00–2:30 p.m.	
2:30–3:00 p.m.	
3:00–3:30 p.m.	
3:30–4:00 p.m.	
4:00–4:30 p.m.	
4:30–5:00 p.m.	
5:00–5:30 p.m.	
5:30–6:00 p.m.	
6:00–6:30 p.m.	
6:30–7:00 p.m.	
7:00–7:30 p.m.	
7:30–8:00 p.m.	
8:00–8:30 p.m.	
8:30–9:00 p.m.	
9:00–9:30 p.m.	
9:30–10:00 p.m.	
10:00–10:30 p.m.	
10:30–11:00 p.m.	
11:00–11:30 p.m.	
11:30 p.m.–12:00 a.m.	

Step #2: List all of the activities for the week in the template, and calculate the total time spent per activity. Decide whether the activity is required or whether you can shift your time spent on this activity to more purposeful tasks. For required activities, consider how you might reduce your time spent on the activity.

ACTIVITY	TOTAL TIME (WEEKDAY)	TOTAL TIME (WEEKEND DAY)	CAN YOU REPURPOSE THIS FOR MORE CONSCIOUS LIVING? HOW?

FIND THE SILVER LINING WORKSHEET

Use this worksheet as a template to practice finding the good in situations that may otherwise cause you, or a family member, to feel negative emotions such as sadness, disappointment, frustration, or anger. Find opportunities to take action to address the challenge now, or prevent it from occurring again in the future.

A COMMON CHALLENGE (OR MISFORTUNE) THAT I'VE FACED IS . . .	A POSITIVE OUTCOME OF THIS ISSUE IS . . .	AN ACTION I COULD TAKE TO ADDRESS THIS CHALLENGE INCLUDES . . .
My classmates did not invite me to join them at the movie theatre.	I got to spend time with my family at the museum and met a new friend.	Share my disappointment with friends and ask to be included next time.

REFRAME NEGATIVE SELF-TALK
WORKSHEET

Use this worksheet as a template to counter negative self-talk with positive, uplift-
ing comments that you can repeat to yourself. Go one step further by thinking about
how it makes you feel to compliment yourself—track these words and feelings in the
appropriate section.

NEGATIVE, SELF-DEFEATING THOUGHT	POSITIVE, UPLIFTING THOUGHT

How does it feel to say something positive about yourself? Choose five to ten words to describe your emotions.

How can you shift your thinking so that positive thoughts are more frequent?

NOTES

Introduction

1. Lally, P., Van Jaarsveld, C. H., Potts, H. W., & Wardle, J. (2010). How are habits formed: Modelling habit formation in the real world. *European Journal of Social Psychology, 40(6),* 998–1009.

2. Hill, J. O. (2009). Can a small-changes approach help address the obesity epidemic? A report of the Joint Task Force of the American Society for Nutrition, Institute of Food Technologists, and International Food Information Council. *American Journal of Clinical Nutrition, 89(2),* 477–484.

3. Pew Research Center. (2015, December 17). *Parenting in America: Outlook, worries, aspirations are strongly linked to financial situation.* Retrieved from http://www .pewsocialtrends.org/2015/12/17/parenting-in-america/.

Week 1: Tickle Your Funny Bone

1. Manninen, S., Tuominen, L., Dunbar, R., Karjalainen, T., Hirvonen, J., Arponen, E., . . . Nummenmaa, L. (2017). Social laughter triggers endogenous opioid release in humans. *Journal of Neuroscience,* 0688–16.

2. Berk, L. S., Tan, S. A., Fry, W. F., Napier, B. J., Lee, J. W., Hubbard, R. W., . . . Eby, W. C. (1989). Neuroendocrine and stress hormone changes during mirthful laughter. *American Journal of the Medical Sciences, 298(6),* 390–396.

3. Clark, A., Seidler, A., & Miller, M. (2001). Inverse association between sense of humor and coronary heart disease. *International Journal of Cardiology, 80(1),* 87–88.

4. Vlachopoulos, C., Xaplanteris, P., Alexopoulos, N., Aznaouridis, K., Vasiliadou, C., Baou, K., . . . Stefanadis, C. (2009). Divergent effects of laughter and mental stress on arterial stiffness and central hemodynamics. *Psychosomatic Medicine, 71(4),* 446–453.

5. Hayashi, K., Kawachi, I., Ohira, T., Kondo, K., Shirai, K., & Kondo, N. (2016). Laughter is the best medicine? A cross-sectional study of cardiovascular disease among older Japanese adults. *Journal of Epidemiology, 26(10),* 546–552.

6. Hayashi, T., Tsujii, S., Iburi, T., Tamanaha, T., Yamagami, K., Ishibashi, R., . . . Murakami, K. (2007). Laughter up-regulates the genes related to NK cell activity in diabetes. *Biomedical Research, 28(6),* 281–285.

7. Sakai, Y., Takayanagi, K., Ohno, M., Inose, R., & Fujiwara, H. (2013). A trial of improvement of immunity in cancer patients by laughter therapy. *Japan-Hospitals, 32,* 53–59.

8. Romundstad, S., Svebak, S., Holen, A., & Holmen, J. (2016). A 15-year follow-up study of sense of humor and causes of mortality: The Nord-Trøndelag Health Study. *Psychosomatic Medicine, 78(3),* 345–353.

9. Manninen, S., Tuominen, L., Dunbar, R., Karjalainen, T., Hirvonen, J., Arponen, E., . . . Nummenmaa, L. (2017). Social laughter triggers endogenous opioid release in humans. *Journal of Neuroscience*, 0688–16.

10. Caird, S., & Martin, R. A. (2014). Relationship-focused humor styles and relationship satisfaction in dating couples: A repeated-measures design. *Humor*, 27(2), 227–247.

11. Martin, R., & Kuiper, N. A. (2016). Three decades investigating humor and laughter: An interview with Professor Rod Martin. *Europe's Journal of Psychology*, 12(3), 498.

Week 2: Sleep Soundly

1. Division of Sleep Medicine, Harvard Medical School. (2007, December 18). *Natural patterns of sleep.* Retrieved from http://healthysleep.med.harvard.edu/healthy/science/what/sleep-patterns-rem-nrem.

2. Faraut, B., Boudjeltia, K. Z., Vanhamme, L., & Kerkhofs, M. (2012). Immune, inflammatory and cardiovascular consequences of sleep restriction and recovery. *Sleep Medicine Reviews*, 16(2), 137–149.

3. Jones, J. M. (2013, December 19). In U.S., 40 percent gets less than recommended amount of sleep. Well-Being, *Gallup News*. Retrieved from http://news.gallup.com/poll/166553/less-recommended-amount-sleep.aspx.

4. Keyes, K. M., Maslowsky, J., Hamilton, A., & Schulenberg, J. (2015). The great sleep recession: Changes in sleep duration among US adolescents, 1991–2012. *Pediatrics*, 135(3), 460–468.

5. Beebe, D. W. (2011). Cognitive, behavioral, and functional consequences of inadequate sleep in children and adolescents. *Pediatric Clinics of North America*, 58(3), 649–665. http://doi.org/10.1016/j.pcl.2011.03.002.

6. Wong, M. M., Brower, K. J., & Zucker, R. A. (2009). Childhood sleep problems, early onset of substance use and behavioral problems in adolescence. *Sleep Medicine*, 10(7), 787–796. http://doi.org/10.1016/j.sleep.2008.06.015.

7. Gregory, A. M., Van der Ende, J., Willis, T. A., & Verhulst, F. C. (2008). Parent-reported sleep problems during development and self-reported anxiety/depression, attention problems, and aggressive behavior later in life. *Archives of Pediatrics & Adolescent Medicine*, 162(4), 330–335.

8. Gregory, A. M., Eley, T. C., O'Connor, T. G., & Plomin, R. (2004). Etiologies of associations between childhood sleep and behavioral problems in a large twin sample. *Journal of the American Academy of Child & Adolescent Psychiatry*, 43(6), 744–751.

9. Roane, B. M., & Taylor, D. J. (2008). Adolescent insomnia as a risk factor for early adult depression and substance abuse. *Sleep*, 31(10), 1351–1356.

10. O'Brien, E. M., & Mindell, J. A. (2005). Sleep and risk-taking behavior in adolescents. *Behavioral Sleep Medicine*, 3(3), 113–133.

11. Altevogt, B. M., & Colten, H. R. (Eds.). (2006). *Sleep disorders and sleep deprivation: An unmet public health problem.* Washington, DC: National Academies Press.

12. Rea, C. J., Smith, R. L., & Taveras, E. M. (2016). Associations of parent health behaviors and parenting practices with sleep duration in overweight and obese children. *Journal of Clinical Sleep Medicine, 12*(11), 1493.

13. Heid, M. (2016, July 19). What's the best time to sleep? You asked. Health, *Time*. Retrieved from http://time.com/3183183/you-asked-whats-the-ideal-time -to-go-to-sleep/.

14. Hirshkowitz, M., Whiton, K., Albert, S. M., Alessi, C., Bruni, O., DonCarlos, L., . . . Neubauer, D. N. (2015). National Sleep Foundation's sleep time duration recommendations: Methodology and results summary. *Sleep Health, 1*(1), 40–43.

15. Ibid.

16. Mustian, K. M. (2013). Yoga as treatment for insomnia among cancer patients and survivors: A systematic review. *European Medical Journal. Oncology 1*, 106–115.

17. Uchida, S., Shioda, K., Morita, Y., Kubota, C., Ganeko, M., & Takeda, N. (2012). Exercise effects on sleep physiology. *Frontiers in Neurology, 3*, 48.

18. Brand, S., Kalak, N., Gerber, M., Kirov, R., Pühse, U., & Holsboer-Trachsler, E. (2014). High self-perceived exercise exertion before bedtime is associated with greater objectively assessed sleep efficiency. *Sleep Medicine, 15*(9), 1031–1036.

19. El-Sohemy, A., Cornelis, M. C., Kabagambe, E. K., & Campos, H. (2007). Coffee, CYP1A2 genotype and risk of myocardial infarction. *Genes & Nutrition, 2*(1), 155–156.

Week 3: Hydrate Healthfully

1. Jéquier, E., & Constant, F. (2010). Water as an essential nutrient: The physiological basis of hydration. *European Journal of Clinical Nutrition, 64*(2), 115–123.

2. EFSA Panel on Dietetic Products, Nutrition and Allergies (NDA). (2011). Scientific opinion on the substantiation of health claims related to water and maintenance of normal physical and cognitive function (ID 1102, 1209, 1294, 1331), maintenance of normal thermoregulation (ID 1208) and "basic requirement of all living things" (ID 1207) pursuant to Article 13(1) of Regulation (EC) No 1924/2006. *EFSA Journal, 9*(4), 2075.

3. Shanley, L., Mittal, V., & Flores, G. (2013). Preventing dehydration-related hospitalizations: A mixed-methods study of parents, inpatient attendings, and primary care physicians. *Hospital Pediatrics, 3*(3), 204–211.

4. Goodman, A. B., Blanck, H. M., Sherry, B., Park, S., Nebeling, L., & Yaroch, A. L. (2013). Peer reviewed: Behaviors and attitudes associated with low drinking water intake among US adults, food attitudes and behaviors survey, 2007. *Preventing Chronic Disease, 10*.

5. National Hydration Council. (2016, September 1). *Drink as I do: The influence of parents' drink choices on children*. Retrieved from http://www.naturalhydrationcouncil .org.uk/press/drink-as-i-do/.

6. Academy of Nutrition and Dietetics. (2017, May 2). *Water: How much do kids need?* Retrieved from http://www.eatright.org/resource/fitness/sports-and-performance /hydrate-right/water-go-with-the-flow.

7. European Hydration Institute. (2014, September 2). *Assessing hydration status.* Retrieved from http://www.europeanhydrationinstitute.org/human-hydration /assessing-hydration-status/

8. American Heart Association. (2016, August 22). *Children should eat less than 25 grams of added sugars daily.* Retrieved from http://newsroom.heart.org/news/children-should -eat-less-than-25-grams-of-added-sugars-daily.

9. Mayo Clinic. (n.d.). *Dehydration signs and symptoms.* Retrieved from http://www .mayoclinic.org/diseases-conditions/dehydration/symptoms-causes/dxc-20261072 on 6/13/17.

Week 4: Be a Bookworm

1. Reading "Can Help Reduce Stress." (2009, March 30). *Telegraph.* Retrieved from http:// www.telegraph.co.uk/news/health/news/5070874/Reading-can-help-reduce-stress .html.

2. National Center for Education Statistics. (2013). *The nation's report card: Trends in academic progress 2012 (NCES 2013–456).* National Center for Education Statistics, Institute of Education Sciences, U.S. Department of Education, Washington, DC. Retrieved from http://nces.ed.gov/nationsreportcard/.

3. Hutton, J. S., Horowitz-Kraus, T., Mendelsohn, A. L., DeWitt, T., Holland, S. K., & C-MIND Authorship Consortium. (2015). Home reading environment and brain activation in preschool children listening to stories. *Pediatrics, 136*(3), 466–478.

4. Massaro, D. W. (2015). Two different communication genres and implications for vocabulary development and learning to read. *Journal of Literacy Research, 47*(4), 505–527.

5. Sticht, T. G. (2011). Getting it right from the start: The case for early parenthood education. *American Educator, 35*(3), 35–39.

6. Scholastic. (2016). *Kids and family reading report* (6th ed.). Retrieved from http://www .scholastic.com/readingreport/files/Scholastic-KFRR-6ed-2017.pdf.

7. Marchessault, J. K., & Larwin, K. H. (2013). Structured read-aloud in middle school: The potential impact on reading achievement. *Contemporary Issues in Education Research* (online), *6*(2), 241.

8. Scholastic. (2013). *Kids and family reading report: 4th edition.* Retrieved from http:// mediaroom.scholastic.com/kfrr.

9. Ibid.

10. Ibid.

11. See note 6 above.

12. See note 6 above.

Week 5: Minimize and Organize

1. McMains, S., & Kastner, S. (2011). Interactions of top-down and bottom-up mechanisms in human visual cortex. *Journal of Neuroscience, 31*(2), 587–597. http://doi.org/10.1523/JNEUROSCI.3766-10.2011.

2. Arnold, J. E., Graesch, A. P., Ragazzini, E., & Ochs, E. (2012). *Life at home in the twenty-first century: 32 families open their doors.* Los Angeles, CA: Cotsen Institute of Archaeology Press.

3. Dush, C. M. K., Schmeer, K. K., & Taylor, M. (2013). Chaos as a social determinant of child health: Reciprocal associations? *Social Science & Medicine, 95,* 69–76.

4. Eller, K. (2016, June 6). *Health benefits of a clean house.* Retrieved from http://www.ahchealthenews.com/2016/06/06/staying-fit-cleaning-house/.

5. Johnson, A. D., Martin, A., Brooks-Gunn, J., & Petrill, S. A. (2008). Order in the house! Associations among household chaos, the home literacy environment, maternal reading ability, and children's early reading. *Merrill-Palmer Quarterly* (Wayne State University Press), *54*(4), 445.

6. See note 2 above.

Week 6: Befriend the Sun

1. Martineau, A. R., Cates, C. J., Urashima, M., Jensen, M., Griffiths, A. P., Nurmatov, U., . . . Griffiths, C. J. (2016). Vitamin D for the management of asthma. *Cochrane Database of Systematic Reviews, 8*(CD011511). doi:10.1002/14651858.CD011511.pub2.

2. Penckofer, S., Kouba, J., Byrn, M., & Ferrans, C. E. (2010). Vitamin D and depression: Where is all the sunshine? *Issues in Mental Health Nursing, 31*(6), 385–393. http://doi.org/10.3109/01612840903437657.

3. OSU Linus Pauling Institute, Micronutrient Information Center. (2014, July). *Vitamin D.* Retrieved from http://lpi.oregonstate.edu/mic/vitamins/vitamin-D.

4. Mansbach, J. M., Ginde, A. A., & Camargo, C. A. (2009). Serum 25-Hydroxyvitamin D levels among US children aged 1 to 11 years: Do children need more vitamin D? *Pediatrics, 124*(5), 1404–1410. http://doi.org/10.1542/peds.2008-2041.

5. Gropper, S. S., & Smith, J. L. (2012). *Advanced nutrition and human metabolism.* Cengage Learning, 392.

6. Vitamin D Council. (2013, December 10). *Why does the Vitamin D Council recommend 5,000 IU/day?* Retrieved from https://www.vitamindcouncil.org/why-does-the-vitamin-d-council-recommend-5000-iuday/.

7. Vitamin D Council. (n.d.). *How do I get the vitamin D my body needs?* Retrieved from https://www.vitamindcouncil.org/about-vitamin-d/how-do-i-get-the-vitamin-d-my-body-needs/.

8. Kimball, S. M., Mirhosseini, N., & Holick, M. F. (2017). Evaluation of vitamin D3 intakes up to 15,000 international units/day and serum 25-hydroxyvitamin D

concentrations up to 300 nmol/L on calcium metabolism in a community setting. *Dermato-Endocrinology, 9*(1), e1300213.

9. Vitamin D Council. (n.d.). *Vitamin D during pregnancy and lactation.* Retrieved from https://www.vitamindcouncil.org/vitamin-d-during-pregnancy-and-breastfeeding.

10. Matsuoka, L. Y., Ide, L., Wortsman, J., MacLaughlin, J. A., & Holick, M. F. (1987). Sunscreens suppress cutaneous vitamin D3 synthesis. *Journal of Clinical Endocrinology and Metabolism, 64,* 1165–8.

11. Environmental Working Group. (n.d.). *What's wrong with high SPF?* Retrieved from http://www.ewg.org/sunscreen/report/whats-wrong-with-high-spf/.

12. Ibid.

Week 7: Foster a Positive Relationship to Food

1. Ellyn Satter Institute. (n.d.). The Satter eating competence model (ecSatter). Retrieved from http://www.ellynsatterinstitute.org/other/ecsatter.php.

2. Satter, E. M. (2007). Eating competence: definition and evidence for the Satter Eating Competence Model. *Journal of Nutrition Education and Behavior, 39,* S142-S153.

3. Christian, M. S., Evans, C. E., Hancock, N., Nykjaer, C., & Cade, J. E. (2013). Family meals can help children reach their 5 a day: A cross-sectional survey of children's dietary intake from London primary schools. *Journal of Epidemiology and Community Health, 67*(4), 332–338.

4. Birch, L. L., Zimmerman, S. I., & Hind, H. (1980). The influence of social-affective context on the formation of children's food preferences. *Child Development,* 856–861.

5. Birch, L. L., Marlin, D. W., & Rotter, J. (1984). Eating as the "means" activity in a contingency: Effects on young children's food preference. *Child Development,* 431–439.

6. Newman, J., & Taylor, A. (1992). Effect of a means-end contingency on young children's food preferences. *Journal of Experimental Child Psychology, 53*(2), 200–216.

7. Gorton's Seafood. *Make a meal of it.* Retrieved from https://www.gortons.com/making-a-meal-of-it/.

8. Kelder, S. H., Perry, C. L., Klepp, K. I., & Lytle, L. L. (1994). Longitudinal tracking of adolescent smoking, physical activity, and food choice behaviors. *American Journal of Public Health, 84*(7), 1121–1126.

9. Abramovitz, B. A., & Birch, L. L. (2000). Five-year-old girls' ideas about dieting are predicted by their mothers' dieting. *Journal of the American Dietetic Association, 100*(10), 1157–1163. Retrieved from http://doi.org/10.1016/S0002-8223(00)00339-4.

10. Hill, A. J., Weaver, C., & Blundell, J. E. (1990). Dieting concerns of 10-year-old girls and their mothers. *British Journal of Clinical Psychology, 29*(3), 346–348.

11. Jarman, M., Ogden, J., Inskip, H., Lawrence, W., Baird, J., Cooper, C., . . . Barker, M. (2015). How do mothers manage their preschool children's eating habits and does this change as children grow older? A longitudinal analysis. *Appetite, 95,* 466–474.

12. Musick, K., & Meier, A. (2012). Assessing causality and persistence in associations between family dinners and adolescent well-being. *Journal of Marriage and the Family, 74*(3), 476–493.

13. Meier, A., & Musick, K. (2014). Variation in associations between family dinners and adolescent well-being. *Journal of Marriage and the Family, 76*(1), 13–23. http://doi .org/10.1111/jomf.12079.

14. Harrison, M. E., Norris, M. L., Obeid, N., Fu, M., Weinstangel, H., & Sampson, M. (2015). Systematic review of the effects of family meal frequency on psychosocial outcomes in youth. *Canadian Family Physician, 61*(2), e96–e106.

15. The Center for Mindful Eating. (n.d.). *Introducing mindful eating.* Retrieved from https://www.thecenterformindfuleating.org/IntroMindfulEating.

Week 8: Make Screen Time Purposeful

1. Swing, E. L., Gentile, D. A., Anderson, C. A., & Walsh, D. A. (2010). Television and video game exposure and the development of attention problems. *Pediatrics, 126*(2), 214–221.

2. Lillard, A. S., & Peterson, J. (2011). The immediate impact of different types of television on young children's executive function. *Pediatrics, 128*(4), 644–649.

3. Martin, K. (2011). Electronic overload: The impact of excessive screen use on child and adolescent health and well-being. Perth, Western Australia: Department of Sport and Recreation.

4. Christakis, D. A., Zimmerman, F. J., DiGiuseppe, D. L., & McCarty, C. A. (2004). Early television exposure and subsequent attentional problems in children. *Pediatrics, 113*(4), 708–713.

5. Kaiser Family Foundation Study. (2010, January 1). *Generation M2: Media in the lives of 8- to 18-year-olds.* Retrieved from https://www.kff.org/other/poll-finding/ report-generation-m2-media-in-the-lives/.

6. Thomée, S. (2012). ICT use and mental health in young adults: Effects of computer and mobile phone use on stress, sleep disturbances, and symptoms of depression. University of Gothenburg.

7. See note 3 above.

8. De Jong, E., Visscher, T. L. S., HiraSing, R. A., Heymans, M. W., Seidell, J. C., & Renders, C. M. (2013). Association between TV viewing, computer use and overweight, determinants and competing activities of screen time in 4- to 13-year-old children. *International Journal of Obesity, 37*(1), 47–53.

9. Richards, R., McGee, R., Williams, S. M., Welch, D., & Hancox, R. J. (2010). Adolescent screen time and attachment to parents and peers. *Archives of Pediatrics & Adolescent Medicine, 164*(3), 258–262.

10. Clements, R. (2004). An investigation of the states of outdoor play. *Contemporary Issues in Early Childhood, 5* (1), 68–80.

11. Tandon, P. S., Zhou, C., Lozano, P., & Christakis, D. A. (2011). Preschoolers' total daily screen time at home and by type of child care. *Journal of Pediatrics*, 158(2), 297–300.

12. Hill, D., Ameenuddin, N., Chassiakos, Y. L. R., Cross, C., Hutchinson, J., Levine, A., . . . Swanson, W. S. (2016). Media and young minds. *Pediatrics*, e20162591.

13. Hill, D., Ameenuddin, N., Chassiakos, Y. L. R., Cross, C., Radesky, J., Hutchinson, J., . . . Swanson, W. S. (2016). Media use in school-aged children and adolescents. *Pediatrics*, e20162592.

14. Vik, F. N., Bjørnarå, H. B., Øverby, N. C., Lien, N., Androutsos, O., Maes, L., . . . Manios, Y. (2013). Associations between eating meals, watching TV while eating meals and weight status among children, ages 10–12 years in eight European countries: The ENERGY cross-sectional study. *International Journal of Behavioral Nutrition and Physical Activity*, 10(1), 58.

Week 9: Say Thanks

1. Froh, J. J., Emmons, R. A., Card, N. A., Bono, G., & Wilson, J. A. (2011). Gratitude and the reduced costs of materialism in adolescents. *Journal of Happiness Studies*, 12(2), 289–302.

2. Froh, J. J., Bono, G., Fan, J., Emmons, R. A., Henderson, K., Harris, C., . . . Wood, A. M. (2014). Nice thinking! An educational intervention that teaches children to think gratefully. *School Psychology Review*, 43(2), 132.

3. Mojtabai, R., Olfson, M., & Han, B. (2016). National trends in the prevalence and treatment of depression in adolescents and young adults. *Pediatrics*, e20161878.

4. Wood, A. M., Joseph, S., Lloyd, J., & Atkins, S. (2009). Gratitude influences sleep through the mechanism of pre-sleep cognitions. *Journal of Psychosomatic Research*, 66(1), 43–48.

5. Wood, A. M., Maltby, J., Gillett, R., Linley, P. A., & Joseph, S. (2008). The role of gratitude in the development of social support, stress, and depression: Two longitudinal studies. *Journal of Research in Personality*, 42(4), 854–871.

6. Bartlett, M. Y., & DeSteno, D. (2006). Gratitude and prosocial behavior: Helping when it costs you. *Psychological Science*, 17(4), 319–325.

7. Froh, J. J., Bono, G., & Emmons, R. (2010). Being grateful is beyond good manners: Gratitude and motivation to contribute to society among early adolescents. *Motivation and Emotion*, 34(2), 144–157.

8. Campbell, E. (2016, November 8). *Three activities to help students deepen their gratitude*. Retrieved from http://greatergood.berkeley.edu/article/item/three_activities _to_help_students_deepen_their_gratitude.

9. See note 2 above.

Week 10: Bust a Move

1. Centers for Disease Control. (2015, June 4). *Physical activity and health.* Retrieved from https://www.cdc.gov/physicalactivity/basics/pa-health/index.htm.

2. Janssen, X., Basterfield, L., Parkinson, K. N., Pearce, M., Reilly, J. K., Adamson, A. J., & Reilly, J. J. (2015). Determinants of changes in sedentary time and breaks in sedentary time among 9 and 12 year old children. *Preventive Medicine Reports, 2*, 880–885.

3. Liu, M., Wu, L., & Ming, Q. (2015). How does physical activity intervention improve self-esteem and self-concept in children and adolescents? Evidence from a meta-analysis. *PloS One,* 10(8), e0134804.

4. Zahl, T., Steinsbekk, S., & Wichstrøm, L. (2017). Physical activity, sedentary behavior, and symptoms of major depression in middle childhood. *Pediatrics,* e20161711.

5. Zecevic, C. A., Tremblay, L., Lovsin, T., & Michel, L. (2010). Parental influence on young children's physical activity. *International Journal of Pediatrics, 2010.* https://www.hindawi.com/journals/ijpedi/2010/468526/.

6. Hesketh, K. R., Goodfellow, L., Ekelund, U., McMinn, A. M., Godfrey, K. M., Inskip, H. M., . . . van Sluijs, E. M. (2014). Activity levels in mothers and their preschool children. *Pediatrics,* 133(4), e973-e980. http://pediatrics.aappublications.org/content/pediatrics/133/4/e973.full.pdf.

7. Scudder, M. R., Federmeier, K. D., Raine, L. B., Direito, A., Boyd, J. K., & Hillman, C. H. (2014). The association between aerobic fitness and language processing in children: Implications for academic achievement. *Brain and Cognition,* 87, 140–152.

8. Smith, L., Gardner, B., Aggio, D., & Hamer, M. (2015). Association between participation in outdoor play and sport at 10 years old with physical activity in adulthood. *Preventive Medicine,* 74, 31–35.

9. Zhang, J., Brackbill, D., Yang, S., & Centola, D. (2015). Efficacy and causal mechanism of an online social media intervention to increase physical activity: Results of a randomized controlled trial. *Preventive Medicine Reports, 2*, 651–657.

10. Sirriyeh, R., Lawton, R., & Ward, J. (2010). Physical activity and adolescents: An exploratory randomized controlled trial investigating the influence of affective and instrumental text messages. *British Journal of Health Psychology,* 15(4), 825–840.

Week 11: Eat the Rainbow

1. Moore, L. V., & Thompson, F. E. (2015). Adults meeting fruit and vegetable intake recommendations—United States, 2013. *Morbidity and Mortality Weekly Report,* 64(26), 709–713.

2. Oyebode, O., Gordon-Dseagu, V., Walker, A., & Mindell, J. S. (2014). Fruit and vegetable consumption and all-cause, cancer and CVD mortality: Analysis of Health Survey for England data. *Journal of Epidemiology and Community Health,* jech-2013.

3. Hung, H. C., Joshipura, K. J., Jiang, R., Hu, F. B., Hunter, D., Smith-Warner, S. A., . . . Willett, W. C. (2004). Fruit and vegetable intake and risk of major chronic disease. *Journal of the National Cancer Institute, 96*(21), 1577–1584.

4. Gee, L. C., & Ahluwalia, A. (2016). Dietary nitrate lowers blood pressure: Epidemiological, pre-clinical experimental and clinical trial evidence. *Current Hypertension Reports, 18*(2), 1–14.

5. Kapil, V., Khambata, R. S., Robertson, A., Caulfield, M. J., & Ahluwalia, A. (2015). Dietary nitrate provides sustained blood pressure lowering in hypertensive patients. *Hypertension, 65*(2), 320–327.

6. Lidder, S., & Webb, A. J. (2013). Vascular effects of dietary nitrate (as found in green leafy vegetables and beetroot) via the nitrate-nitrite-nitric oxide pathway. *British Journal of Clinical Pharmacology, 75*(3), 677–696. http://doi.org/10.1111 /j.1365-2125.2012.04420.x.

7. Webb, A. J., Patel, N., Loukogeorgakis, S., Okorie, M., Aboud, Z., Misra, S., . . . MacAllister, R. (2008). Acute blood pressure lowering, vasoprotective, and antiplatelet properties of dietary nitrate via bioconversion to nitrite. *Hypertension, 51*(3), 784–790.

8. Krebs-Smith, S. M., Reedy, J., & Bosire, C. (2010). Healthfulness of the U.S. food supply: Little improvement despite decades of dietary guidance. *American Journal of Preventive Medicine, 38*(5), 472–477. http://doi.org/10.1016/j.amepre.2010.01.016.

Week 12: Just Breathe

1. Clarke, T. C., Black, L. I., Stussman, B. J., Barnes, P. M., & Nahin, R. L. (2015). Trends in the use of complementary health approaches among adults: United States, 2002–2012. *National Health Statistics Reports,* (79), 1.

2. Black, L. I., Clarke, T. C., Barnes, P. M., Stussman, B. J., & Nahin, R. L. (2015). Use of complementary health approaches among children aged 4–17 years in the United States: National Health Interview Survey, 2007–2012. *National Health Statistics Reports,* (78), 1.

3. Goyal, M., Singh, S., Sibinga, E. M., Gould, N. F., Rowland-Seymour, A., Sharma, R., . . . Ranasinghe, P. D. (2014). Meditation programs for psychological stress and well-being: A systematic review and meta-analysis. *JAMA Internal Medicine, 174*(3), 357–368.

4. Black, D. S., & Slavich, G. M. (2016). Mindfulness meditation and the immune system: A systematic review of randomized controlled trials. *Annals of the New York Academy of Sciences, 1373*(1), 13–24.

5. Flook, L., Smalley, S. L., Kitil, M. J., Galla, B. M., Kaiser-Greenland, S., Locke, J., . . . Kasari, C. (2010). Effects of mindful awareness practices on executive functions in elementary school children. *Journal of Applied School Psychology, 26*(1), 70–95.

6. Black et al. (2015). Use of complementary health approaches among children.

7. Hölzel, B. K., Carmody, J., Vangel, M., Congleton, C., Yerramsetti, S. M., Gard, T., & Lazar, S. W. (2011). Mindfulness practice leads to increases in regional brain gray matter density. *Psychiatry Research: Neuroimaging, 191*(1), 36–43.

8. Fox, K. C., Nijeboer, S., Dixon, M. L., Floman, J. L., Ellamil, M., Rumak, S. P., . . . Christoff, K. (2014). Is meditation associated with altered brain structure? A systematic review and meta-analysis of morphometric neuroimaging in meditation practitioners. *Neuroscience & Biobehavioral Reviews, 43*, 48–73.

Week 13: Let Your Imagination Run Wild

1. Stuckey, H. L., & Nobel, J. (2010). The connection between art, healing, and public health: A review of current literature. *American Journal of Public Health, 100*(2), 254–263. http://doi.org/10.2105/AJPH.2008.156497.

2. McFadden, S. H., & Basting, A. D. (2010). Healthy aging persons and their brains: Promoting resilience through creative engagement. *Clinics in Geriatric Medicine, 26*(1), 149–161.

3. Beebe, A., Gelfand, E. W., & Bender, B. (2010). A randomized trial to test the effectiveness of art therapy for children with asthma. *Journal of Allergy and Clinical Immunology, 126*(2), 263–266.

4. Americans for the Arts. (Updated April 2015). Improved academic performance for students with high level of arts involvement. Retrieved on 6/15/17.

5. World Economic Forum. (2016, January 18). *The future of jobs: Employment, skills and workforce strategy for the fourth industrial revolution.* Retrieved from https://www .weforum.org/reports/the-future-of-jobs.

Week 14: Set Goals

1. Locke, E. A., & Latham, G. P. (2006). New directions in goal-setting theory. *Current Directions in Psychological Science, 15*(5), 265–268.

2. Northwestern Mutual. (2015). *Planning and progress study.* Retrieved from https:// www.northwesternmutual.com/about-us/studies/planning-and-progress-2015-study.

3. National Council on Aging. (2013). *The United States of aging survey.* Retrieved from http://www.bgaaail.org/docs/AOA percent20Survey.pdf.

4. Statistic Brain Research Institute. (2017). *New year's resolution statistics.* Retrieved from http://www.statisticbrain.com/new-years-resolution-statistics.

5. Morisano, D., Hirsh, J. B., Peterson, J. B., Pihl, R. O., & Shore, B. M. (2010). Setting, elaborating, and reflecting on personal goals improves academic performance. *Journal of Applied Psychology, 95*(2), 255.

6. Clark, D., Gill, D., Prowse, V., & Rush, M. (2017). *Using Goals To Motivate College Students: Theory and Evidence From Field Experiments* (No. w23638). National Bureau of Economic Research.

7. Pruitt, S. (2015, December 30). *The history of new year's resolutions.* Retrieved from http://www.history.com/news/the-history-of-new-years-resolutions.

Week 15: Know Your Farmer

1. Ramberg, J., & McAnalley, B. (2002). From the farm to the kitchen table: A review of the nutrient losses in foods. *GlycoScience & Nutrition, 3*(5), 1–12.

2. Pew Charitable Trust and Robert Wood Johnson Foundation. (2016, December). *School meal programs innovate to improve school nutrition.* Retrieved from http://www.pewtrusts.org/en/research-and-analysis/reports/2016/12/school-meal-programs-innovate-to-improve-student-nutrition.

3. Yoder, A. B. B., Liebhart, J. L., McCarty, D. J., Meinen, A., Schoeller, D., Vargas, C., & LaRowe, T. (2014). Farm to elementary school programming increases access to fruits and vegetables and increases their consumption among those with low intake. *Journal of Nutrition Education and Behavior, 46*(5), 341–349.

4. Izumi, B. T., Eckhardt, C. L., Hallman, J. A., Herro, K., & Barberis, D. A. (2015). Harvest for healthy kids pilot study: Associations between exposure to a farm-to-preschool intervention and willingness to try and liking of target fruits and vegetables among low-income children in Head Start. *Journal of the Academy of Nutrition and Dietetics, 115*(12), 2003–2013.

5. Jones, S. J., Childers, C., Weaver, A. T., & Ball, J. (2015). SC farm-to-school programs encourages children to consume vegetables. *Journal of Hunger & Environmental Nutrition, 10*(4), 511–525.

6. Center for Agroecology and Sustainable Food Systems. (2003). *Community supported agriculture: The CSA member experience.* Retrieved from https://casfs.ucsc.edu/documents/research-briefs/RB_1_CSA_members_survey.pdf.

7. Pevec, I. S. (2011). A healthy harvest: Adolescents grow food and well-being with policy implications for education, health and community planning. (Doctoral thesis, University of Colorado at Denver).

8. Runyon, L. (2015, February 5). *Are farmers market sales peaking? That might be good for farmers.* Retrieved from http://www.npr.org/sections/thesalt/2015/02/05/384058943/are-farmer-market-sales-peaking-that-might-be-good-for-farmers.

9. Knowwhereyourfoodcomesfrom.com (n.d.). Dining. Retrieved from http://knowwhereyourfoodcomesfrom.com/farm-to-table-dining/dining/.

10. EarthBox Container gardening system. Retrieved from https://earthbox.com/earthbox-systems/the-original-earthbox-gardening-system.

Week 16: Be a Good Friend

1. Waldinger, R. (2015, December 23). *Robert Waldinger: What makes a good life? Lessons from the longest study on happiness* [Video]. Retrieved from https://www.ted.com/talks/robert_waldinger_what_makes_a_good_life_lessons_from_the_longest_study_on_happiness.

2. Umberson, D., & Karas Montez, J. (2010). Social relationships and health: A flash-point for health policy. *Journal of Health and Social Behavior, 51*(1_suppl), S54–S66.

3. Mineo, L. (2017, April 11). *Good genes are nice, but joy is better.* Retrieved from https://news.harvard.edu/gazette/story/2017/04/over-nearly-80-years-harvard-study-has-been-showing-how-to-live-a-healthy-and-happy-life/.

4. Adams, R. E., Santo, J. B., & Bukowski, W. M. (2011). The presence of a best friend buffers the effects of negative experiences. *Developmental Psychology, 47*(6), 1786.

5. James, B. D., Wilson, R. S., Barnes, L. L., & Bennett, D. A. (2011). Late-life social activity and cognitive decline in old age. *Journal of the International Neuropsychological Society, 17*(6), 998–1005.

Week 17: Smell the Aroma

1. Lee, Y. L., Wu, Y., Tsang, H. W., Leung, A. Y., & Cheung, W. M. (2011). A systematic review on the anxiolytic effects of aromatherapy in people with anxiety symptoms. *Journal of Alternative and Complementary Medicine, 17*(2), 101–108.

2. Hwang, E., & Shin, S. (2015). The effects of aromatherapy on sleep improvement: A systematic literature review and meta-analysis. *Journal of Alternative and Complementary Medicine, 21*(2), 61–68.

3. Jafarzadeh, M., Arman, S., & Pour, F. F. (2013). Effect of aromatherapy with orange essential oil on salivary cortisol and pulse rate in children during dental treatment: A randomized controlled clinical trial. *Advanced Biomedical Research, 2*, 10. http://doi.org/10.4103/2277-9175.107968.

4. Ibid.

5. Neal's Yard Remedies. (n.d.). *Essential oils.* Retrieved from https://us.nyrorganic.com/shop/corp/area/essential-oils/.

6. Maia, M. F., & Moore, S. J. (2011). Plant-based insect repellents: A review of their efficacy, development and testing. *Malaria Journal, 10*(Suppl 1), S11. http://doi.org/10.1186/1475-2875-10-S1-S11.

7. *Essential oils natural remedies: The complete A-Z reference of essential oils for health and healing.* (2015). Althea Press. Emeryville, CA: Callisto Media.

Week 18: Explore Nature

1. Kardan, O., Gozdyra, P., Misic, B., Moola, F., Palmer, L. J., Paus, T., & Berman, M. G. (2015). Neighborhood greenspace and health in a large urban center. *Scientific Reports, 5*, 11610.

2. Donovan, G. H., Butry, D. T., Michael, Y. L., Prestemon, J. P., Liebhold, A. M., Gatziolis, D., & Mao, M. Y. (2013). The relationship between trees and human health: Evidence from the spread of the emerald ash borer. *American Journal of Preventive Medicine, 44*(2), 139–145.

3. Thompson, C. W., Roe, J., Aspinall, P., Mitchell, R., Clow, A., & Miller, D. (2012). More green space is linked to less stress in deprived communities: Evidence from salivary cortisol patterns. *Landscape and Urban Planning, 105*(3), 221–229.

4. Bratman, G. N., Daily, G. C., Levy, B. J., & Gross, J. J. (2015). The benefits of nature experience: Improved affect and cognition. *Landscape and Urban Planning, 138*, 41–50.

5. Charles, C., & Wheeler, K. (2012). Children & nature worldwide: An exploration of children's experiences of the outdoors and nature with associated risks and benefits. Children and Nature Network and the IUCN's Commission on Education and Communication.

6. Taylor, A. F., Kuo, F. E., & Sullivan, W. C. (2001). Coping with ADD: The surprising connection to green play settings. *Environment and Behavior, 33*(1), 54–77.

7. Juster, F. T., Ono, H., & Stafford, F. P. (2004, November). Changing times of American youth: 1981–2003. *Institute for Social Research*, 1–15.

8. Tandon, P. S., Zhou, C., & Christakis, D. A. (2012). Frequency of parent-supervised outdoor play of US preschool-aged children. *Archives of Pediatrics & Adolescent Medicine, 166*(8), 707–712.

9. Tandon, P. S., Zhou, C., Lozano, P., & Christakis, D. A. (2011). Preschoolers' total daily screen time at home and by type of child care. *Journal of Pediatrics, 158*(2), 297–300.

10. Institute for Communications Technology Management. (2013). *How much media? 2013 report on American consumers*. Retrieved from https://business.tivo.com/content /dam/tivo/resources/tivo-HMM-Consumer-Report-2013_Release.pdf.

11. Park, B. J., Tsunetsugu, Y., Kasetani, T., Kagawa, T., & Miyazaki, Y. (2010). The physiological effects of *Shinrin-yoku* (taking in the forest atmosphere or forest bathing): Evidence from field experiments in 24 forests across Japan. *Environmental Health and Preventive Medicine, 15*(1), 18–26. http://doi.org/10.1007/s12199-009-0086-9.

12. Kardan, O., Gozdyra, P., Misic, B., Moola, F., Palmer, L. J., Paus, T., & Berman, M. G. (2015). Neighborhood greenspace and health in a large urban center. *Scientific Reports, 5*, 11610.

Week 19: Choose Grains Wisely

1. Whole Grains Council. (2015, August 31). *Survey: Two thirds of Americans make half their grains whole*. Retrieved from https://wholegrainscouncil.org/blog/2015/08 /survey-two-thirds-americans-make-half-their-grains-whole.

2. Foster-Powell, K., Holt, S. H., & Brand-Miller, J. C. (2002). International table of glycemic index and glycemic load values: 2002. *American Journal of Clinical Nutrition, 76*(1), 5–56.

3. Benisi-Kohansal, S., Saneei, P., Salehi-Marzijarani, M., Larijani, B., & Esmaillzadeh, A. (2016). Whole-grain intake and mortality from all causes, cardiovascular disease, and cancer: A systematic review and dose-response meta-analysis of prospective cohort studies. *Advances in Nutrition: An International Review Journal, 7*(6), 1052–1065.

4. de Munter, J. S., Hu, F. B., Spiegelman, D., Franz, M., & van Dam, R. M. (2007). Whole grain, bran, and germ intake and risk of type 2 diabetes: A prospective cohort study and systematic review. *PLoS Med*, 4(8), e261.

5. Harris, L. A., Hansel, S., DiBaise, J., & Crowell, M. D. (2006). Irritable bowel syndrome and chronic constipation: Emerging drugs, devices, and surgical treatments. *Current Gastroenterology Reports*, 8(4), 282–290.

6. Whole Grain Council. (2017). *Whole grain stamp.* Retrieved from https://wholegrainscouncil.org/whole-grain-stamp.

7. Leonard, M. M., & Vasagar, B. (2014). US perspective on gluten-related diseases. *Clinical and Experimental Gastroenterology*, 7, 25–37. http://doi.org/10.2147/CEG.S54567.

8. De Punder, K., & Pruimboom, L. (2013). The dietary intake of wheat and other cereal grains and their role in inflammation. *Nutrients*, 5(3), 771–787. http://doi.org/10.3390/nu5030771.

9. Zevallos, V. F., Raker, V., Tenzer, S., Jimenez-Calvente, C., Ashfaq-Khan, M., Rüssel, N., . . . Schuppan, D. (2017). Nutritional wheat amylase-trypsin inhibitors promote intestinal inflammation via activation of myeloid cells. *Gastroenterology*, 152(5), 1100–1113.

10. Kresser, C. (2017, May 24). Is gluten killing your brain? Kresser Institute for Functional and Evolutionary Training. https://kresserinstitute.com/gluten-killing-brain/.

11. United European Gastroenterology. (2016, October 17). UEG Week: New study links protein in wheat to the inflammation of chronic health conditions [Press release]. Retrieved from https://www.ueg.eu/press/releases/ueg-press-release/article/new-study-links-protein-in-wheat-to-the-inflammation-of-chronic-health-conditions/.

12. Ibid.

13. Schuppan, D., Pickert, G., Ashfaq-Khan, M., & Zevallos, V. (2015). Non-celiac wheat sensitivity: Differential diagnosis, triggers and implications. *Best Practice & Research Clinical Gastroenterology*, 29(3), 469–476.

14. Zevallos, V. F., Raker, V., Tenzer, S., Jimenez-Calvente, C., Ashfaq-Khan, M., Rüssel, N., . . . Schuppan, D. (2017). Nutritional wheat amylase-trypsin inhibitors promote intestinal inflammation via activation of myeloid cells. *Gastroenterology*, 152(5), 1100–1113.

Week 20: Heal with Touch

1. Ardiel, E. L., & Rankin, C. H. (2010). The importance of touch in development. *Paediatrics & Child Health*, 15(3), 153–156.

2. Silva, L. M., Schalock, M., Gabrielsen, K. R., Budden, S. S., Buenrostro, M., & Horton, G. (2015). Early intervention with a parent-delivered massage protocol directed at tactile abnormalities decreases severity of autism and improves child-to-parent interactions: A replication study. *Autism Research and Treatment*, 2015.

3. Field, T., Hernandez-Reif, M., Hart, S., Theakston, H., Schanberg, S., & Kuhn, C. (1999). Pregnant women benefit from massage therapy. *Journal of Psychosomatic Obstetrics & Gynecology, 20*(1), 31–38.

4. Harris, M., Richards, K. C., & Grando, V. T. (2012). The effects of slow-stroke back massage on minutes of nighttime sleep in persons with dementia and sleep disturbances in the nursing home: A pilot study. *Journal of Holistic Nursing, 30*(4), 255–263.

5. Olff, M., Frijling, J. L., Kubzansky, L. D., Bradley, B., Ellenbogen, M. A., Cardoso, C., . . . van Zuiden, M. (2013). The role of oxytocin in social bonding, stress regulation and mental health: An update on the moderating effects of context and interindividual differences. *Psychoneuroendocrinology, 38*(9), 1883–1894.

6. Paloyelis, Y., Krahé, C., Maltezos, S., Williams, S. C., Howard, M. A., & Fotopoulou, A. (2016). The analgesic effect of oxytocin in humans: A double-blind, placebo-controlled cross-over study using laser-evoked potentials. *Journal of Neuroendocrinology, 28*(4).

7. Light, K. C., Grewen, K. M., & Amico, J. A. (2005). More frequent partner hugs and higher oxytocin levels are linked to lower blood pressure and heart rate in premenopausal women. *Biological Psychology, 69*(1), 5–21.

8. Gürol, A., & Polat, S. (2012). The effects of baby massage on attachment between mother and their infants. *Asian Nursing Research, 6*(1), 35–41.

9. Kraus, M. W., Huang, C., & Keltner, D. (2010). Tactile communication, cooperation, and performance: An ethological study of the NBA. *Emotion, 10*(5), 745.

10. Rapaport, M. H., Schettler, P., & Bresee, C. (2012). A preliminary study of the effects of repeated massage on hypothalamic–pituitary–adrenal and immune function in healthy individuals: A study of mechanisms of action and dosage. *Journal of Alternative and Complementary Medicine, 18*(8), 789–797.

Week 21: Discover Your True North

1. Making Caring Common, Harvard Graduate School of Education. (2014). *The children we mean to raise.* Retrieved from https://mcc.gse.harvard.edu/the-children -we-mean-to-raise.

2.Parker, K. (2014, September 18). *Families may differ, but they share common values on parenting.* FactTank, Pew Research Center. Retrieved from http://www.pewresearch.org/ fact-tank/2014/09/18/families-may-differ-but-they-share-common-values-on -parenting/.

Week 22: Turn on the Tunes

1. Bradt, J., & Dileo, C. (2009). Music for stress and anxiety reduction in coronary heart disease patients. *The Cochrane Database of Systematic Reviews, 2*(1).

2. Stefano, G. B., Zhu, W., Cadet, P., Salamon, E., & Mantione, K. J. (2004). Music alters constitutively expressed opiate and cytokine processes in listeners. *Medical Science Monitor, 10*(6), MS18–MS27.

3. Bottiroli, S., Rosi, A., Russo, R., Vecchi, T., & Cavallini, E. (2014). The cognitive effects of listening to background music on older adults: Processing speed improves with upbeat music, while memory seems to benefit from both upbeat and downbeat music. *Frontiers in Aging Neuroscience, 6*, 284.

4. Zhao, T. C., & Kuhl, P. K. (2016). Musical intervention enhances infants' neural processing of temporal structure in music and speech. *Proceedings of the National Academy of Sciences*, 201603984.

5. Van de Carr, R., & Lehrer, M. (1986). Enhancing early speech, parental bonding and infant physical development using prenatal intervention in standard obstetric practice. *Journal of Prenatal & Perinatal Psychology & Health, 1*(1).

6. Bugos, J. A., Perlstein, W. M., McCrae, C. S., Brophy, T. S., & Bedenbaugh, P. H. (2007). Individualized piano instruction enhances executive functioning and working memory in older adults. *Aging and Mental Health, 11*(4), 464–471.

7. Wong, P. C., Chan, A. H., Roy, A., & Margulis, E. H. (2011). The bimusical brain is not two monomusical brains in one: Evidence from musical affective processing. *Journal of Cognitive Neuroscience, 23*(12), 4082–4093.

8. Brown, L. L. (n.d.). *What music should my children listen to?* Education, PBS Parents. Retrieved from http://www.pbs.org/parents/education/music-arts/what-music-should -my-child-listen-to/ on 6/14/17.

9. Hanser, S. B., & Mandel, S. E. (2010). *Manage your stress and pain through music.* Boston, MA: Berklee Press.

Week 23: Be a Conscious Carnivore

1. Environmental Protection Agency. (n.d.) *Animal feeding operations (AFOs)*. Retrieved from https://www.epa.gov/npdes/animal-feeding-operations-afos on 7/15/17.

2. Environmental Protection Agency. (2004). *Risk assessment evaluation for concentrated animal feeding operations*. Retrieved from https://www.epa.gov/npdes/animal-feeding -operations-afos#AFO on 7/15/17.

3. Sapkota, A. R., Lefferts, L. Y., McKenzie, S., & Walker, P. (2007). What do we feed to food-production animals? A review of animal feed ingredients and their potential impacts on human health. *Environmental Health Perspectives, 115*(5), 663–670. http://doi .org/10.1289/ehp.9760.

4. Nachman, K. E., Baron, P. A., Raber, G., Francesconi, K. A., Navas-Acien, A., & Love, D. C. (2013). Roxarsone, inorganic arsenic, and other arsenic species in chicken: A U.S.-based market basket sample. *Environmental Health Perspectives, 121*(7), 818–824. http://doi.org/10.1289/ehp.1206245.

5. European Commission. (n.d.). *Hormones in meat*. Retrieved from https://ec.europa.eu /food/safety/chemical_safety/meat_hormones_en.

6. Liou, A. P., & Turnbaugh, P. J. (2012). Antibiotic exposure promotes fat gain. *Cell Metabolism, 16*(4), 408–410. http://doi.org/10.1016/j.cmet.2012.09.009.

7. Siemon, C. E., Bahnson, P. B., & Gebreyes, W. A. (2007). Comparative investigation of prevalence and antimicrobial resistance of *Salmonella* between pasture and conventionally reared poultry. *Avian Diseases, 51*(1), 112–117.

8. Eamens, G. J., Hornitzky, M. A., Walker, K. H., Hum, S. I., Vanselow, B. A., Bailey, G. D., . . . Gill, P. A. (2003). A study of the foodborne pathogens: *Campylobacter, Listeria* and *Yersinia* in faeces from slaughter-age cattle and sheep in Australia. *Communicable Diseases Intelligence Quarterly Report, 27*(2), 249.

9. Gallup. (2013). *Frequency of family dining, according to U.S. parents.* Retrieved from http://www.gallup.com/poll/166628/families-routinely-dine-together-home.aspx.

10. Pew Charitable Trusts. (2012, July 18). *How corporate control squeezes out small farms.* Retrieved from http://www.pewtrusts.org/en/research-and-analysis/fact-sheets /2012/07/18/how-corporate-control-squeezes-out-small-farms.

11. National Bison Association. (n.d.). *Ranchers' commitment to responsible bison production.* Retrieved from https://bisoncentral.com/husbandry-item /ranchers-commitment-to-responsible-bison-production/.

Week 24: Toss Plastics

1. Kay, V. R., Bloom, M. S., & Foster, W. G. (2014). Reproductive and developmental effects of phthalate diesters in males. *Critical Reviews in Toxicology, 44*(6), 467–498.

2. Poursafa, P., Ataei, E., & Kelishadi, R. (2015). A systematic review on the effects of environmental exposure to some organohalogens and phthalates on early puberty. *Journal of Research in Medical Sciences 20*(6), 613–618. http://doi.org /10.4103/1735-1995.165971.

3. Rochester, J. R., & Bolden, A. L. (2015). Bisphenol S and F: A systematic review and comparison of the hormonal activity of bisphenol A substitutes. *Environmental Health Perspectives, 123*(7), 643.

4. Yang, C. Z., Yaniger, S. I., Jordan, V. C., Klein, D. J., & Bittner, G. D. (2011). Most plastic products release estrogenic chemicals: A potential health problem that can be solved. *Environmental Health Perspectives, 119*(7), 989–996. http://doi.org/10.1289 /ehp.1003220.

5. Westervelt, A. (2015, February 10). Phthalates are everywhere, and the health risks are worrying. How bad are they really? *Guardian.* Retrieved from https://www .theguardian.com/lifeandstyle/2015/feb/10phthalates-plastics-chemicals -research-analysis.

6. EWG Action Fund. (2015). *Tests find asbestos in kids' crayons, crime scene kits.* Retrieved from http://www.asbestosnation.org/facts/tests-find-asbestos -in-kids-crayons-crime-scene-kits/#fullreport.

7. Environmental Working Group. (2015, May 1). *Poisoned legacy.* Retrieved from http:// www.ewg.org/research/poisoned-legacy/executive-summary.

Week 25: Have Real Conversations

1. Konrath, S. H., O'Brien, E. H., & Hsing, C. (2011). Changes in dispositional empathy in American college students over time: A meta-analysis. *Personality and Social Psychology Review, 15*(2), 180–198.

2. The Children's Society. (2013). *The good childhood report 2013.* Retrieved from https://www.childrenssociety.org.uk/sites/default/files/tcs/good_childhood_report_2013_final.pdf.

3. Hacker, K. A., Amare, Y., Strunk, N., & Horst, L. (2000). Listening to youth: Teen perspectives on pregnancy prevention. *Journal of Adolescent Health, 26*(4), 279–288.

4. Martino, S. C., Elliott, M. N., Corona, R., Kanouse, D. E., & Schuster, M. A. (2008). Beyond the "big talk": The roles of breadth and repetition in parent-adolescent communication about sexual topics. *Pediatrics, 121*(3), e612–e618.

5. Chaplin, T. M., Hansen, A., Simmons, J., Mayes, L. C., Hommer, R. E., & Crowley, M. J. (2014). Parental–adolescent drug use discussions: Physiological responses and associated outcomes. *Journal of Adolescent Health, 55*(6), 730–735.

6. Simons-Morton, B., Haynie, D. L., Crump, A. D., Eitel, P., & Saylor, K. E. (2001). Peer and parent influences on smoking and drinking among early adolescents. *Health Education & Behavior, 28*(1), 95–107.

7. PayScale Human Capital. (2016). *2016 workforce-skills preparedness report.* Retrieved from http://www.payscale.com/data-packages/job-skills.

8. Pew Research Center. (2015, August 26). *Americans' views on mobile etiquette.* Retrieved from http://www.pewinternet.org/files/2015/08/2015-08-26_mobile-etiquette_FINAL.pdf.

9. Turkle, S. (2015, September 26). Stop googling. Let's talk. Sunday Review, *New York Times.* Retrieved from https://www.nytimes.com/2015/09/27/opinion/sunday/stop-googling-lets-talk.html.

Week 26: Nurture Spirituality

1. Gallup. (2016). *Religion.* Retrieved from http://www.gallup.com/poll/1690/religion.aspx.

2. Calculations based on the U.S. Census Bureau's July 2016 Current Population Data, which estimates there are 249,454,440 adults in the U.S.

3. Scales, P. C. (2007, February). *Spirituality and adolescent well-being: Selected new statistics (Fast Fact).* [Research brief].

4. Scales, P. C., Syvertsen, A. K., Benson, P. L., Roehlkepartain, E. C., & Sesma Jr, A. (2014). Relation of spiritual development to youth health and well-being: Evidence from a global study. In A. Ben-Arieh, F. Casas, I. Frones, & J. E. Korbin (Eds.), *Handbook of child well-being*, (2), 1101–1135. Dordrecht, The Netherlands: Springer Netherlands.

5. Siedlecki, K. L., Salthouse, T. A., Oishi, S., & Jeswani, S. (2014). The relationship between social support and subjective well-being across age. *Social Indicators Research*, 117(2), 561–576.

6. Ecklund, E. H., Johnson, D. R., Scheitle, C. P., Matthews, K. R., & Lewis, S. W. (2016). Religion among scientists in international context: A new study of scientists in eight regions. *Socius*, 2, https://doi.org/10.1177/2378023116664353.

7. Gallup. (2017, May 15). *Record few Americans believe bible is literal word of God.* Retrieved from http://www.gallup.com/poll/210704/record-few-americans-believe -bible-literal-word-god.aspx.

8. Miller, L. (2016). *The spiritual child: The new science on parenting for health and lifelong thriving.* New York, NY: Macmillan.

Week 27: Conquer Added Sugar

1. Nguyen, S., Choi, H. K., Lustig, R. H., & Hsu, C. (2009). Sugar sweetened beverages, serum uric acid, and blood pressure in adolescents. *Journal of Pediatrics*, 154(6), 807–813. http://doi.org/10.1016/j.jpeds.2009.01.015.

2. Ibid.

3. Knüppel, A., Shipley, M. J., Llewellyn, C. H., & Brunner, E. J. (2017). Sugar intake from sweet food and beverages, common mental disorder and depression: Prospective findings from the Whitehall II study. *Scientific Reports*, 7.

4. Scragg, R. K., McMichael, A. J., & Baghurst, P. A. (1984). Diet, alcohol, and relative weight in gall stone disease: A case-control study. *British Medical Journal (Clinical Research ed.)*, 288(6424), 1113–1119.

5. Thornley, S., Stewart, A., Marshall, R., & Jackson, R. (2011). Per capita sugar consumption is associated with severe childhood asthma: An ecological study of 53 countries. *Primary Care Respiratory Journal*, 20(1), 75–78.

6. Reinehr, T. (2013). Type 2 diabetes mellitus in children and adolescents. *World Journal of Diabetes*, 4(6), 270–281. http://doi.org/10.4239/wjd.v4.i6.270.

7. Benton, D., Maconie, A., & Williams, C. (2007). The influence of the glycaemic load of breakfast on the behaviour of children in school. *Physiology & Behavior*, 92(4), 717–724.

8. O'Neil, A., Quirk, S. E., Housden, S., Brennan, S. L., Williams, L. J., Pasco, J. A., . . . Jacka, F. N. (2014). Relationship between diet and mental health in children and adolescents: A systematic review. *American Journal of Public Health*, 104(10), e31–e42. http://doi.org/10.2105/AJPH.2014.302110.

9. Steele, E. M., Baraldi, L. G., da Costa Louzada, M. L., Moubarac, J. C., Mozaffarian, D., & Monteiro, C. A. (2016). Ultra-processed foods and added sugars in the US diet: Evidence from a nationally representative cross-sectional study. *BMJ Open*, 6(3), e009892.

10. American Heart Association. (2016, August 22). *Children should eat less than 25 grams of added sugars daily.* Retrieved from http://newsroom.heart.org/news /children-should-eat-less-than-25-grams-of-added-sugars-daily.

11. Kelder, S. H., Perry, C. L., Klepp, K. I., & Lytle, L. L. (1994). Longitudinal tracking of adolescent smoking, physical activity, and food choice behaviors. *American Journal of Public Health, 84*(7), 1121–1126.

12. Savage, J. S., Fisher, J. O., & Birch, L. L. (2007). Parental influence on eating behavior: Conception to adolescence. *Journal of Law, Medicine & Ethics, 35*(1), 22–34. http://doi .org/10.1111/j.1748-720X.2007.00111.x.

13. Videon, T. M., & Manning, C. K. (2003). Influences on adolescent eating patterns: the importance of family meals. *Journal of Adolescent Health, 32*(5), 365–373.

14. U.S. Food and Drug Administration. (n.d.). *Learn about the nutrition facts label.* Retrieved from https://www.accessdata.fda.gov/scripts /InteractiveNutritionFactsLabel/#intro.

15. See note 9 above.

16. Schmitz, A. (Ed.). (2002). *Sugar and related sweetener markets: International perspectives.* Wallingford, Oxfordshire, UK: Centre for Agriculture and Biosciences International (CABI).

17. Ahmed, S. H., Guillem, K., & Vandaele, Y. (2013). Sugar addiction: Pushing the drug-sugar analogy to the limit. *Current Opinion in Clinical Nutrition & Metabolic Care, 16*(4), 434–439.

18. Harvard Medical School. (2016, December 12). *Artificial sweeteners: Sugar-free, but at what cost?* Retrieved from https://www.health.harvard.edu/blog/artificial-sweeteners -sugar-free-but-at-what-cost-201207165030.

19. Environmental Working Group. (2014). *Children's cereals: Sugar by the pound.* Washington, DC: Environmental Working Group.

Week 28: Love to Do, Not to Have

1. Van Boven, L., & Gilovich, T. (2003). To do or to have? That is the question. *Journal of Personality and Social Psychology, 85*(6), 1193.

2. Caprariello, P. A., & Reis, H. T. (2013). To do, to have, or to share? Valuing experiences over material possessions depends on the involvement of others. *Journal of Personality and Social Psychology, 104*(2), 199.

3. University of California Television. (n.d.). *University of California TV series looks at clutter epidemic in middle-class American homes.* Retrieved from http://www.uctv.tv /RelatedContent.aspx?RelatedID=301.

4. Maslow, A. H. (1943). A theory of human motivation. *Psychological Review, 50*(4), 370.

Week 29: Surf and Socialize Online Safely

1. Erickson, T. (2012, April 18). How mobile technologies are shaping a new generation. *Harvard Business Review.*

2. Common Sense Media. (2013). *Zero to eight: Children's media use in America 2013.* Retrieved from https://www.commonsensemedia.org/research/zero-to-eight-childrens-media-use-in-america-2013.

3. Pew Research Center. (2015, April 9). *Teens, social media & technology overview 2015: Smartphones facilitate shifts in communication landscape for teens.* Retrieved from http://www.pewinternet.org/2015/04/09/teens-social-media-technology-2015/.

4. Pew Research Center. (2016, November 6). *Mobile fact sheet.* Retrieved from http://www.pewinternet.org/fact-sheet/mobile/.

5. Livingstone, S., & Smith, P. K. (2014). Annual research review: Harms experienced by child users of online and mobile technologies: The nature, prevalence and management of sexual and aggressive risks in the digital age. *Journal of Child Psychology and Psychiatry, 55*(6), 635–654.

6. Collins, R. L., Martino, S., & Shaw, R. (2010). *Influence of new media on adolescent sexual health* (Working Paper WR-761). Santa Monica, CA: Rand Health.

7. The Henry J. Kaiser Family Foundation. (2005, February 27). *Generation M: Media in the lives of 8–18 year-olds – Report.* Retrieved from http://www.kff.org/other/generation-m-media-in-the-lives-of/.

8. See note 6 above.

9. Javelin Strategy & Research. (2017, February 1). *2017 identify fraud study.* Retrieved from https://www.javelinstrategy.com/press-release/identity-fraud-hits-record-high-154-million-us-victims-2016-16-percent-according-new.

10. Power, R. (2011). *Child identity theft: New evidence indicates identity thieves are targeting children for unused Social Security numbers.* Carnegie Mellon CyLab.

11. EU Kids Online (2014). *EU Kids Online: Findings, methods, recommendations.* EU Kids Online, LSE. http://eprints.lse.ac.uk/60512/.

12. Mobile Media Guard. (n.d.). *U.S. sexting laws.* Retrieved from http://mobilemediaguard.com/state_main.html.

13. Pew Research Center. (2015, August 6). *Teens, technology & friendships.* Retrieved from http://www.pewinternet.org/2015/08/06/teens-technology-and-friendships/.

14. MediaSmarts. (n.d.). *Internet safety tips by age.* Retrieved from http://mediasmarts.ca.

Week 30: Love Your Body

1. Common Sense Media. (2015, January 21). *Children, teens, media and body image.* Retrieved from https://www.commonsensemedia.org/research/children-teens-media-and-body-image.

2. National Eating Disorders Association. (n.d.). *What are eating disorders?* Retrieved from https://www.nationaleatingdisorders.org/get-facts-eating-disorders.

3. Record, K. L., & Austin, S. B. (2016). "Paris Thin": A call to regulate life-threatening starvation of runway models in the US fashion industry.

4. Nota, B. (2013, January 3). *Israeli law bans skinny, BMI-challenged models*. Retrieved from http://abcnews.go.com/International/israeli-law-bans-skinny-bmi-challenged -models/story?id=18116291.

5. BBC. (2017, May 6). *France bans extremely thin models*. Retrieved from http://www.bbc .com/news/world-europe-39821036.

6. Eisenberg, M. E., Wall, M., & Neumark-Sztainer, D. (2012). Muscle-enhancing behaviors among adolescent girls and boys. *Pediatrics*, peds-2012.

7. Field, A. E., Sonneville, K. R., Crosby, R. D., Swanson, S. A., Eddy, K. T., Camargo, C. A., . . . Micali, N. (2014). Prospective associations of concerns about physique and the development of obesity, binge drinking, and drug use among adolescent boys and young adult men. *JAMA Pediatrics*, 168(1), 34–39.

8. Swanson, S. A., Crow, S. J., Le Grange, D., Swendsen, J., & Merikangas, K. R. (2011). Prevalence and correlates of eating disorders in adolescents: Results from the national comorbidity survey replication adolescent supplement. *Archives of General Psychiatry*, 68(7), 714–723.

Week 31: Go Fish

1. Kalmijn, S. V., Van Boxtel, M. P. J., Ocke, M., Verschuren, W. M. M., Kromhout, D., & Launer, L. J. (2004). Dietary intake of fatty acids and fish in relation to cognitive performance at middle age. *Neurology*, 62(2), 275–280.

2. Chung, W. L., Chen, J. J., & Su, H. M. (2008). Fish oil supplementation of control and (n-3) fatty acid-deficient male rats enhances reference and working memory performance and increases brain regional docosahexaenoic acid levels. *Journal of Nutrition*, 138(6), 1165–1171.

3. National Marine Fisheries Service, Office of Science and Technology. (September 2016). *Fisheries of the United States, Current Fishery Statistics 2015*. Retrieved from http:// www.st.nmfs.noaa.gov/commercial-fisheries/fus/fus15/index.

4. Oken, E., Radesky, J. S., Wright, R. O., Bellinger, D. C., Amarasiriwardena, C. J., Kleinman, K. P., . . . Gillman, M. W. (2008). Maternal fish intake during pregnancy, blood mercury levels, and child cognition at age 3 years in a US cohort. *American Journal of Epidemiology*, 167(10), 1171–1181.

5. Silbernagel, S. M., Carpenter, D. O., Gilbert, S. G., Gochfeld, M., Groth, E., Hightower, J. M., & Schiavone, F. M. (2011). Recognizing and preventing overexposure to methylmercury from fish and seafood consumption: Information for physicians. *Journal of Toxicology*, 2011, 983072. http://doi.org/10.1155/2011/983072.

6. Easton, M. D. L., Luszniak, D., & Von der Geest, E. (2002). Preliminary examination of contaminant loadings in farmed salmon, wild salmon and commercial salmon feed. *Chemosphere*, 46(7), 1053–1074.

7. Environmental Working Group. (2014). EWG releases new consumer tool to help people make smarter seafood choices [Press release]. Retrieved from https://www.ewg.org/release/ewg-releases-new-consumer-tool-help-people-make-smarter-seafood-choices#.Whi0fWeAnF8.

Week 32: Respect Differences

1. United Nations, Department of Economic and Social Affairs, Population Division (2016). International Migration Report 2015: Highlights (ST/ESA/SER.A/375).

2. Pew Research Center. (2016, March 31). 10 demographic trends that are shaping the U.S. and the world. http://www.pewresearch.org/fact-tank/2016/03/31/10-demographic-trends-that-are-shaping-the-u-s-and-the-world/.

3. Gallup. (2017, January 11). In US, more adults identifying as LGBT. http://www.gallup.com/poll/201731/lgbt-identification-rises.aspx.

4. Barak, M., & Levenberg, A. (2016). Flexible thinking in learning: An individual differences measure for learning in technology-enhanced environments. Computers & Education, 99, 39–52.

5. Hayes, S. C., Luoma, J. B., Bond, F. W., Masuda, A., & Lillis, J. (2006). Acceptance and commitment therapy: Model, processes and outcomes. Behaviour Research and Therapy, 44(1), 1–25.

6. Kashdan, T. B., & Rottenberg, J. (2010). Psychological flexibility as a fundamental aspect of health. Clinical Psychology Review, 30(7), 865–878.

7. See note 5 above.

8. Martínez-Martí, M. L., & Ruch, W. (2014). Character strengths and well-being across the life span: Data from a representative sample of German-speaking adults living in Switzerland. Frontiers in Psychology, 5, 1253. http://doi.org/10.3389/fpsyg.2014.01253.

9. Richard, O., McMillan, A., Chadwick, K., & Dwyer, S. (2003). Employing an innovation strategy in racially diverse workforces: Effects on firm performance. Group & Organization Management, 28(1), 107–126.

10. Bassett-Jones, N. (2005). The paradox of diversity management, creativity and innovation. Creativity and Innovation Management, 14(2), 169–175.

11. Kreitz, C., Schnuerch, R., Gibbons, H., & Memmert, D. (2015). Some see it, some don't: Exploring the relation between inattentional blindness and personality factors. PloS One, 10(5), e0128158.

12. Kelly, D. J., Quinn, P. C., Slater, A. M., Lee, K., Gibson, A., Smith, M., . . . Pascalis, O. (2005). Three-month-olds, but not newborns, prefer own-race faces. Developmental Science, 8(6), F31–F36. http://doi.org/10.1111/j.1467-7687.2005.0434a.x.

13. Metzler, C. (2009). Teaching children about diversity. PBS Parents. http://www.pbs.org/parents/experts/archive/2009/02/teaching-children-about-divers.html.

14. Reischer, E. (2017, February 23). 3 essentials for parents in turbulent times [Web log post, 2nd item]. Retrieved from http://www.drericar.com/blog/.

Week 33: Go Beyond the Piggy Bank

1. Bridges, S., & Disney, R. (2010). Debt and depression. *Journal of Health Economics, 29*(3), 388–403.

2. Sweet, E., Nandi, A., Adam, E., & McDade, T. (2013). The high price of debt: Household financial debt and its impact on mental and physical health. *Social Science & Medicine, 91,* 94–100. http://doi.org/10.1016/j.socscimed.2013.05.009.

3. Federal Reserve Bank of New York. (May 2017). *Quarterly report on household debt and credit.* Retrieved from https://www.newyorkfed.org/microeconomics/hhdc.html.

4. Brown, A. M., Collins, J. M., Schmeiser, M. D., & Urban, C. (2014). *State mandated financial education and the credit behavior of young adults.* Retrieved from http://www.finrafoundation.org/.

5. Kim, J., & Chatterjee, S. (2013). Childhood financial socialization and young adults' financial management. *Journal of Financial Counseling and Planning, 24*(1), 61.

6. Mottola, G. R. (2014, March). The financial capability of young adults—A generational view. *Insights: Financial Capability.*

Week 34: Push the Boundaries

1. Gross, J., & Rosin, H. (2014, August 6). The shortening leash. *Slate.* Retrieved from http://www.slate.com/articles/life/family/2014/08/slate_childhood_survey_results_kids_today_have_a_lot_less_freedom_than_their.2.html.

2. Ingraham, C. (2015, April 14). There's never been a safer time to be a kid in America. *Washington Post.*

3. Biswas-Diener, R., & Kashdan, T. B. (2013, July 2). What happy people do differently. *Psychology Today.* Retrieved from https://www.psychologytoday.com/articles/201307/what-happy-people-do-differently.

4. Sandseter, E. B. H., & Kennair, L. E. O. (2011). Children's risky play from an evolutionary perspective: The anti-phobic effects of thrilling experiences. *Evolutionary Psychology, 9*(2), https://doi.org/10.1177/147470491100900212.

5. Poulton, R., Davies, S., Menzies, R. G., Langley, J. D., & Silva, P. A. (1998). Evidence for a non-associative model of the acquisition of a fear of heights. *Behaviour Research and Therapy, 36*(5), 537–544.

6. Rosin, H. (2014, April). The overprotected kid. *Atlantic.* Retrieved from https://www.theatlantic.com/magazine/archive/2014/04/hey-parents-leave-those-kids-alone/358631/.

7. Green, J. (1997). Risk and the construction of social identity: Children's talk about accidents. *Sociology of Health & Illness, 19*(4), 457–479.

8. Gerber, M., & Johnson, A. (2002). *Your self-confident baby: How to encourage your child's natural abilities from the very start.* New York, NY: Wiley.

Week 35: Skip the Additives

1. Environmental Working Group. (2014, November 12). *EWG's dirty dozen guide to food additives.* Retrieved from http://www.ewg.org/research/ewg-s-dirty-dozen-guide -food-additives.

2. Jeong, S. H., Kim, B. Y., Kang, H. G., Ku, H. O., & Cho, J. H. (2005). Effects of butylated hydroxyanisole on the development and functions of reproductive system in rats. *Toxicology, 208*(1), 49–62.

3. Oishi, S. (2002). Effects of propyl paraben on the male reproductive system. *Food and Chemical Toxicology, 40*(12), 1807–1813.

4. Okubo, T., Yokoyama, Y., Kano, K., & Kano, I. (2001). ER-dependent estrogenic activity of parabens assessed by proliferation of human breast cancer MCF-7 cells and expression of ERα and PR. *Food and Chemical Toxicology, 39*(12), 1225–1232.

5. Smith, K. W., Souter, I., Dimitriadis, I., Ehrlich, S., Williams, P. L., Calafat, A. M., & Hauser, R. (2013). Urinary paraben concentrations and ovarian aging among women from a fertility center. *Environmental Health Perspectives, 121*(11-12), 1299.

6. Neltner, T. G., Alger, H. M., O'Reilly, J. T., Krimsky, S., Bero, L. A., & Maffini, M. V. (2013). Conflicts of interest in approvals of additives to food determined to be generally recognized as safe: Out of balance. *JAMA Internal Medicine, 173*(22), 2032–2036.

7. Nestle, M. (2013). Conflicts of interest in the regulation of food safety: A threat to scientific integrity. *JAMA Internal Medicine, 173*(22), 2036–2038.

8. American Academy of Pediatrics. (2008). ADHD and food additives revisited. *AAP Grand Rounds, 19*(2), 17.

9. Christian, M. S., Evans, C. E., Hancock, N., Nykjaer, C., & Cade, J. E. (2013). Family meals can help children reach their 5 a day: A cross-sectional survey of children's dietary intake from London primary schools. *Journal of Epidemiology and Community Health, 67*(4), 332–338.

10. Environmental Working Group (2014, October 27). EWG's Food Scores helps people find out what's really in their food [Press release]. https://www.ewg.org/release/ ewg-s-food-scores-helps-people-find-out-what-s-really-their-food.

11. Slusser, W. M., Cumberland, W. G., Browdy, B. L., Lange, L., & Neumann, C. (2007). A school salad bar increases frequency of fruit and vegetable consumption among children living in low-income households. *Public Health Nutrition, 10*(12), 1490–1496.

12. Katz, D. L., Katz, C. S., Treu, J. A., Reynolds, J., Njike, V., Walker, J., . . . Michael, J. (2011). Teaching healthful food choices to elementary school students and their parents: the nutrition detectives program. *Journal of School Health, 81*(1), 21–28.

Week 36: Spread Kindness

1. Ouweneel, E., Le Blanc, P. M., & Schaufeli, W. B. (2014). On being grateful and kind: Results of two randomized controlled trials on study-related emotions and academic engagement. *Journal of Psychology, 148*(1), 37–60.

2. Layous, K., Nelson, S. K., Oberle, E., Schonert-Reichl, K. A., & Lyubomirsky, S. (2012). Kindness counts: Prompting prosocial behavior in preadolescents boosts peer acceptance and well-being. *PLoS One, 7*(12), e51380.

3. Mineo, L. (2017, April 11). Good genes are nice, but joy is better. *Harvard Gazette.* Retrieved from http://news.harvard.edu/gazette/story/2017/04/over-nearly-80-years -harvard-study-has-been-showing-how-to-live-a-healthy-and-happy-life/.

4. Post, S. G. (2011). It's good to be good: 2011 fifth annual scientific report on health, happiness and helping others. *International Journal of Person Centered Medicine, 1*(4), 814–829.

5. Arnstein, P., Vidal, M., Wells-Federman, C., Morgan, B., & Caudill, M. (2002). From chronic pain patient to peer: Benefits and risks of volunteering. *Pain Management Nursing, 3*(3), 94–103.

6. Gutkowska, J., & Jankowski, M. (2012). Oxytocin revisited: Its role in cardiovascular regulation. *Journal of Neuroendocrinology, 24*(4), 599–608.

7. Szeto, A., Nation, D. A., Mendez, A. J., Dominguez-Bendala, J., Brooks, L. G., Schneiderman, N., & McCabe, P. M. (2008). Oxytocin attenuates NADPH-dependent superoxide activity and IL-6 secretion in macrophages and vascular cells. *American Journal of Physiology-Endocrinology and Metabolism, 295*(6), E1495–E1501.

8. Fabes, R. A., Fultz, J., Eisenberg, N., May-Plumlee, T., & Christopher, F. S. (1989). Effects of rewards on children's prosocial motivation: A socialization study. *Developmental Psychology, 25*(4), 509.

9. Chernyak, N., & Kushnir, T. (2013). Giving preschoolers choice increases sharing behavior. *Psychological Science, 24*(10), 1971–1979.

10. Garner, P. W. (2006). Prediction of prosocial and emotional competence from maternal behavior in African American preschoolers. *Cultural Diversity and Ethnic Minority Psychology, 12*(2), 179.

11. Hastings, P. D., McShane, K. E., Parker, R., & Ladha, F. (2007). Ready to make nice: Parental socialization of young sons' and daughters' prosocial behaviors with peers. *Journal of Genetic Psychology, 168*(2), 177–200.

12. Varkey, P., Chutka, D. S., & Lesnick, T. G. (2006). The aging game: Improving medical students' attitudes toward caring for the elderly. *Journal of the American Medical Directors Association, 7*(4), 224–229.

Week 37: Silence the Noise

1. Hammer, M. S., Swinburn, T. K., & Neitzel, R. L. (2014). Environmental noise pollution in the United States: Developing an effective public health response. *Environmental Health Perspectives, 122*(2), 115.

2. Kim, R. (2007). Burden of disease from environmental noise. In Proceedings of the International Workshop on Combined Environmental Exposure: Noise, Air Pollutants and Chemicals, Ispra, Italy.

3. Tiesler, C. M., Birk, M., Thiering, E., Kohlböck, G., Koletzko, S., Bauer, C. P., . . . Heinrich, J. (2013). Exposure to road traffic noise and children's behavioural problems and sleep disturbance: Results from the GINIplus and LISAplus studies. *Environmental Research, 123*, 1–8.

4. Cohen, S., Glass, D. C., & Singer, J. E. (1973). Apartment noise, auditory discrimination, and reading ability in children. *Journal of Experimental Social Psychology, 9*(5), 407–422.

5. Schmidt, M. E., Pempek, T. A., Kirkorian, H. L., Lund, A. F., & Anderson, D. R. (2008). The effects of background television on the toy play behavior of very young children. *Child Development, 79*(4), 1137–1151.

6. Kirkorian, H. L., Pempek, T. A., Murphy, L. A., Schmidt, M. E., & Anderson, D. R. (2009). The impact of background television on parent-child interaction. *Child Development, 80*(5), 1350–1359.

7. Lapierre, M. A., Piotrowski, J. T., & Linebarger, D. L. (2012). Background television in the homes of US children. *Pediatrics, 130*(5), 839–846.

8. Bernardi, L., Porta, C., & Sleight, P. (2006). Cardiovascular, cerebrovascular, and respiratory changes induced by different types of music in musicians and non-musicians: The importance of silence. *Heart, 92*(4), 445–452. http://doi.org/10.1136/hrt.2005.064600.

9. Kirste, I., Nicola, Z., Kronenberg, G., Walker, T. L., Liu, R. C., & Kempermann, G. (2015). Is silence golden? Effects of auditory stimuli and their absence on adult hippocampal neurogenesis. *Brain Structure & Function, 220*(2), 1221–1228. http://doi.org/10.1007/s00429-013-0679-3.

10. See note 1 above.

Week 38: Give Back

1. Thoits, P. A., & Hewitt, L. N. (2001). Volunteer work and well-being. *Journal of Health and Social Behavior*, 115–131.

2. Sneed, R. S., & Cohen, S. (2013). A prospective study of volunteerism and hypertension risk in older adults. *Psychology and Aging, 28*(2), 578.

3. Barak, Y. (2006). The immune system and happiness. *Autoimmunity Reviews, 5*(8), 523–527.

4. Office of Research & Policy Development, Corporation for National & Community Service (US). (2007). *The health benefits of volunteering: A review of recent research.* Retrieved from https://www.nationalservice.gov/pdf/07_0506_hbr.pdf.

5. Sabin, E. P. (1993). Social relationships and mortality among the elderly. *Journal of Applied Gerontology, 12*(1), 44–60.

6. Carlo, G., Crockett, L. J., Wilkinson, J. L., & Beal, S. J. (2011). The longitudinal relationships between rural adolescents' prosocial behaviors and young adult substance use. *Journal of Youth and Adolescence, 40*(9), 1192–1202.

7. Moore, C. W., & Allen, J. P. (1996). The effects of volunteering on the young volunteer. *Journal of Primary Prevention, 17*(2), 231–258.

8. Schreier, H. M., Schonert-Reichl, K. A., & Chen, E. (2013). Effect of volunteering on risk factors for cardiovascular disease in adolescents: A randomized controlled trial. *JAMA Pediatrics, 167*(4), 327–332.

9. Zaff, J. F., & Michelsen, E. (2002). Encouraging civic engagement: How teens are (or are not) becoming responsible citizens. *Child Trends.* Retrieved from https://www.childtrends.org/publications/encouraging-civic-engagement-how-teens-are-or-are-not-becoming-responsible-citizens/.

10. Indiana University Lilly Family School of Philanthropy. (2016, May 19). A tradition of giving: New research on giving and volunteering within families.

11. Aknin, L. B., Hamlin, J. K., & Dunn, E. W. (2012). Giving leads to happiness in young children. *PLoS One, 7*(6), e39211.

12. Grimm Jr., R., Dietz, N., Spring, K., Arey, K., & Foster-Bey, J. (2005). Building active citizens: The role of social institutions in teen volunteering. *Youth Helping America.* Corporation for National and Community Service.

13. Indiana University Lilly Family School of Philanthropy. (2013). *Women give 2013: New research on charitable giving by boys and girls.* Retrieved from https://philanthropy.iupui.edu/files/research/women_give_2013-final9-12-2013.pdf.

14. Weisman, C. E. (2008). *Raising charitable children.* St. Louis, MO: FE Robbins & Sons.

Week 39: Enjoy Healthy Fats

1. Patterson, E., Wall, R., Fitzgerald, G. F., Ross, R. P., & Stanton, C. (2012). Health implications of high dietary omega-6 polyunsaturated fatty acids. *Journal of Nutrition and Metabolism* doi:10.1155/2012/539426.

2. Souza, R. G., Gomes, A. C., Naves, M. M., & Mota, J. F. (2015). Nuts and legume seeds for cardiovascular risk reduction: Scientific evidence and mechanisms of action. *Nutrition Reviews, 73*(6), 335–347.

3. Sprecher, H., Luthria, D. L., Mohammed, B. S., & Baykousheva, S. P. (1995). Reevaluation of the pathways for the biosynthesis of polyunsaturated fatty acids. *Journal of Lipid Research, 36*(12), 2471–2477.

4. Kresser, C. (2016, September 6). An update on Omega-6 PUFAs. Retrieved from https://chriskresser.com/an-update-on-omega-6-pufas/.

5. Chowdhury, R., Warnakula, S., Kunutsor, S., Crowe, F., Ward, H. A., Johnson, L., . . . Khaw, K. T. (2014). Association of dietary, circulating, and supplement fatty acids with coronary risk: A systematic review and meta-analysis. *Annals of Internal Medicine, 160*(6), 398–406.

6. Dreon, D. M., Fernstrom, H. A., Campos, H., Blanche, P., Williams, P. T., & Krauss, R. M. (1998). Change in dietary saturated fat intake is correlated with change in mass of large low-density-lipoprotein particles in men. *American Journal of Clinical Nutrition, 67*(5), 828–836.

7. Hyman, M. (2016, March 30). Fat: What I got wrong, what I got right. Retrieved from http://drhyman.com/blog/2016/03/30/fat-what-i-got-wrong-what-i-got-right/.

8. Sachdeva, A., Cannon, C. P., Deedwania, P. C., LaBresh, K. A., Smith, S. C., Dai, D., . . . Fonarow, G. C. (2009). Lipid levels in patients hospitalized with coronary artery disease: An analysis of 136,905 hospitalizations in Get with the Guidelines [database]. *American Heart Journal, 157*(1), 111–117.

9. Hyman, M. (2016, April 6). Is coconut oil bad for your cholesterol? Retrieved from http://drhyman.com/blog/2016/04/06/is-coconut-oil-bad-for-your-cholesterol/.

Week 40: Clean Up the Chemicals

1. Food and Drug Administration. (Updated March 23, 2014). Cosmetics safety Q&A: Prohibited ingredients. https://www.fda.gov/Cosmetics/ResourcesForYou/Consumers/ucm167234.htm.

2. De Groot, A. C., & Veenstra, M. (2010). Formaldehyde-releasers in cosmetics in the USA and in Europe. *Contact Dermatitis, 62*(4), 221–224.

3. Lefebvre, M. A., Meuling, W. J., Engel, R., Coroama, M. C., Renner, G., Pape, W., & Nohynek, G. J. (2012). Consumer inhalation exposure to formaldehyde from the use of personal care products/cosmetics. *Regulatory Toxicology and Pharmacology, 63*(1), 171–176.

4. Kodjak, A. (2016, September 2). FDA bans 19 chemicals used in antibacterial soaps. Your Health, NPR. Retrieved from http://www.npr.org/sections/health-shots/2016/09/02/492394717/fda-bans-19-chemicals-used-in-antibacterial-soaps.

5. Harley, K. G., Kogut, K., Madrigal, D. S., Cardenas, M., Vera, I. A., Meza-Alfaro, G., . . . Parra, K. L. (2016). Reducing phthalate, paraben, and phenol exposure from personal care products in adolescent girls: Findings from the HERMOSA intervention study. *Environmental Health Perspectives, 124*(10), 1600–1607. http://doi.org/10.1289/ehp.1510514.

6. Grossman, E. (2014, June 9). Banned in Europe, safe in the US. *Ensia*. Retrieved from https://ensia.com/features/banned-in-europe-safe-in-the-u-s/.

7. Summaries of EU Legislation. (2000, February 2). *The precautionary principle*. Retrieved from http://eur-lex.europa.eu/legal-content/EN/TXT/?uri=URISERV percent3Al32042.

8. Kunisue, T., Chen, Z., Buck Louis, G. M., Sundaram, R., Hediger, M. L., Sun, L., & Kannan, K. (2012). Urinary concentrations of benzophenone-type UV filters in US women and their association with endometriosis. *Environmental Science & Technology, 46*(8), 4624–4632.

9. Schlumpf, M., Kypke, K., Wittassek, M., Angerer, J., Mascher, H., Mascher, D., . . . Lichtensteiger, W. (2010). Exposure patterns of UV filters, fragrances, parabens, phthalates, organochlor pesticides, PBDEs, and PCBs in human milk: Correlation of UV filters with use of cosmetics. *Chemosphere, 81*(10), 1171–1183.

10. Louis, G. M. B., Chen, Z., Kim, S., Sapra, K. J., Bae, J., & Kannan, K. (2015). Urinary concentrations of benzophenone-type ultraviolet light filters and semen quality. *Fertility and Sterility, 104*(4), 989–996.

11. Environmental Working Group. (2015, October 19). Duke-EWG study finds toxic nail polish chemical in women's bodies.

12. European Commission. (2005, July 5). *Permanent ban of phthalates: Commission hails long-term safety for children's toys* [Press release]. Retrieved from http://europa.eu/rapid/press-release_IP-05-838_en.htm.

Week 41: Grow Your Mind

1. Gruber, M. J., Gelman, B. D., & Ranganath, C. (2014). States of curiosity modulate hippocampus-dependent learning via the dopaminergic circuit. *Neuron, 84*(2), 486–496.

2. Park, D. C., Lodi-Smith, J., Drew, L., Haber, S., Hebrank, A., Bischof, G. N., & Aamodt, W. (2014). The impact of sustained engagement on cognitive function in older adults: The synapse project. *Psychological Science, 25*(1), 103–112. http://doi.org/10.1177/0956797613499592.

3. Gottfried, A. E., Preston, K. S. J., Gottfried, A. W., Oliver, P. H., Delany, D. E., & Ibrahim, S. M. (2016). Pathways from parental stimulation of children's curiosity to high school science course accomplishments and science career interest and skill. *International Journal of Science Education, 38*(12), 1972–1995.

4. Mindset Works. (n.d.). Teacher practices: How praise and feedback impact student outcomes. Retrieved from https://www.mindsetworks.com/science/Teacher-Practices.

Week 42: Build Inner Strength

1. MacLeod, S., Musich, S., Hawkins, K., Alsgaard, K., & Wicker, E. R. (2016). The impact of resilience among older adults. *Geriatric Nursing, 37*(4), 266–272.

2. Duckworth, A. (2016). *Grit: The power of passion and perseverance.* New York, NY: Simon & Schuster.

3. Zeng, Y., & Shen, K. (2010, December). Resilience significantly contributes to exceptional longevity. *Current Gerontology and Geriatrics Research.* doi: 10.1155/2010/525693.

4. See note 1 above.

5. Werner, E. E. (1995). Resilience in development. *Current Directions in Psychological Science, 4*(3), 81–84.

6. Jobin, J., Wrosch, C., & Scheier, M. F. (2014). Associations between dispositional optimism and diurnal cortisol in a community sample: When stress is perceived as higher than normal. *Health Psychology, 33*(4), 382.

Week 43: Go Organic

1. Office of Health Hazard Assessment, State of California. (2017, June 26). Glyphosate listed effective July 7, 2017, as known to the State of California to cause cancer.

Retrieved from https://oehha.ca.gov/proposition-65/crnr/glyphosate-listed
-effective-july-7-2017-known-state-california-cause-cancer.

2. Lu, C., Toepel, K., Irish, R., Fenske, R. A., Barr, D. B., & Bravo, R. (2006). Organic diets significantly lower children's dietary exposure to organophosphorus pesticides. *Environmental Health Perspectives*, 114(2), 260–263. http://doi.org/10.1289/ehp.8418.

3. Muñoz-Quezada, M. T., Lucero, B. A., Barr, D. B., Steenland, K., Levy, K., Ryan, P. B., . . . Vega, C. (2013). Neurodevelopmental effects in children associated with exposure to organophosphate pesticides: A systematic review. *Neurotoxicology*, 39, 158–168. http://doi.org/10.1016/j.neuro.2013.09.003.

4. Benbrook, C. M., & Baker, B. P. (2014). Perspective on dietary risk assessment of pesticide residues in organic food. *Sustainability*, 6(6), 3552–3570.

5. Ibid.

6. Roberts, J. R., & Karr, C. J. (2012). Pesticide exposure in children. *Pediatrics*, 130(6), e1765-e1788.

7. *Consumer Reports* Food Safety and Sustainability Center. (n.d.). *Natural—not meaningful*. Retrieved from http://greenerchoices.org/2016/11/16/natural-label-review/.

8. See note 6 above.

Week 44: Live Intentionally

1. Killingsworth, M. A., & Gilbert, D. T. (2010). A wandering mind is an unhappy mind. *Science*, 330(6006), 932.

2. Garland, E. L., Froeliger, B., & Howard, M. O. (2013). Mindfulness training targets neurocognitive mechanisms of addiction at the attention-appraisal-emotion interface. *Frontiers in Psychiatry*, 4.

3. Tomfohr, L. M., Pung, M. A., Mills, P. J., & Edwards, K. (2015). Trait mindfulness is associated with blood pressure and interleukin-6: Exploring interactions among subscales of the Five Facet Mindfulness Questionnaire to better understand relationships between mindfulness and health. *Journal of Behavioral Medicine*, 38(1), 28–38.

4. Labelle, L. E., Campbell, T. S., Faris, P., & Carlson, L. E. (2015). Mediators of mindfulness based stress reduction (MBSR): Assessing the timing and sequence of change in cancer patients. *Journal of Clinical Psychology*, 71(1), 21–40.

5. Costa, A., & Barnhofer, T. (2016). Turning towards or turning away: A comparison of mindfulness meditation and guided imagery relaxation in patients with acute depression. *Behavioural and Cognitive Psychotherapy*, 44(4), 410–419.

6. Harpin, S. B., Rossi, A., Kim, A. K., & Swanson, L. M. (2016). Behavioral impacts of a mindfulness pilot intervention for elementary school students. *Education*, 137(2), 149–156.

7. Bennett, K., & Dorjee, D. (2016). The impact of a mindfulness-based stress reduction course (MBSR) on well-being and academic attainment of sixth-form students. *Mindfulness*, 7(1), 105–114.

8. Bureau of Labor Statistics. (2015, June 24). *American time use survey* [News release]. Retrieved from https://www.bls.gov/news.release/archives/atus_06242015.htm.

9. MacLean, K. L. (2009). *Moody cow meditates.* New York, NY: Simon & Schuster.

10. Morris, A. S., Silk, J. S., Steinberg, L., Myers, S. S., & Robinson, L. R. (2007). The role of the family context in the development of emotion regulation. *Social Development, 16*(2), 361–388. http://doi.org/10.1111/j.1467-9507.2007.00389.x.

Week 45: Take Charge of Your Health

1. García, M. C. (2016). Potentially preventable deaths among the five leading causes of death—United States, 2010 and 2014. *Morbidity and Mortality Weekly Report, 65.* Retrieved from https://www.cdc.gov/mmwr/volumes/65/wr/mm6545a1.htm.

2. Pew Research Center. (2014, January 15). *The social life of health information.* Retrieved from http://www.pewresearch.org/fact-tank/2014/01/15/the-social-life-of-health -information/.

3. Stacey, D., Légaré, F., Lewis, K., Barry, M. J., Bennett, C. L., Eden, K. B., . . . Trevena, L. (2017). Decision aids for people facing health treatment or screening decisions. *Cochrane Database of Systematic Reviews.* doi:10.1002/14651858 .CD001431.pub3.

4. Kew, K. M., & Malik, P. (2016). Shared decision-making for people with asthma. *Cochrane Database of Systematic Reviews.* doi:10.1002/14651858.CD012330 .pub2.

5. Coxeter, P., Del Mar, C., McGregor, L., Beller, E., & Hoffmann, T. C. (2015). Interventions to facilitate shared decision making to address antibiotic use for acute respiratory infections in primary care. *Cochrane Database of Systematic Reviews, 11*(CD010907), 1.

6. Tuso, P. (2014). Prediabetes and lifestyle modification: Time to prevent a preventable disease. *Permanente Journal, 18*(3), 88.

7. National Center for Health Statistics. (2017). Health, United States, 2016: With chartbook on long-term trends in health (p. 25, tables 78 and 80).

8. Abramson, J. D., & Redberg, R. F. (2013, November 13). Don't give more patients statins. *New York Times.*

Week 46: Keep on the Sunny Side

1. Gordon, R. A. (2008). Attributional style and athletic performance: Strategic optimism and defensive pessimism. *Psychology of Sport and Exercise, 9*(3), 336–350.

2. Schiavon, C. C., Marchetti, E., Gurgel, L. G., Busnello, F. M., & Reppold, C. T. (2016). Optimism and hope in chronic disease: A systematic review. *Frontiers in Psychology, 7.*

3. DuBois, C. M., Beach, S. R., Kashdan, T. B., Nyer, M. B., Park, E. R., Celano, C. M., & Huffman, J. C. (2012). Positive psychological attributes and cardiac outcomes: Associations, mechanisms, and interventions. *Psychosomatics, 53*(4), 303–318.

4. Conversano, C., Rotondo, A., Lensi, E., Della Vista, O., Arpone, F., & Reda, M. A. (2010). Optimism and its impact on mental and physical well-being. *Clinical Practice and Epidemiology in Mental Health, 6*, 25.

5. Hecht, D. (2013). The neural basis of optimism and pessimism. *Experimental Neurobiology, 22*(3), 173–199.

6. Kleinke, C. L., Peterson, T. R., & Rutledge, T. R. (1998). Effects of self-generated facial expressions on mood. *Journal of Personality and Social Psychology, 74*(1), 272.

Week 47: Cook In, Eat Together

1. *Economist*. (2015, September 14). How countries spend their money. Daily Chart. Retrieved from https://www.economist.com/blogs/graphicdetail/2015/09/daily-chart-9.

2. Smith, L. P., Ng, S. W., & Popkin, B. M. (2013). Trends in US home food preparation and consumption: Analysis of national nutrition surveys and time use studies from 1965–1966 to 2007–2008. *Nutrition Journal, 12*, 45. http://doi.org/10.1186/1475-2891-12-45.

3. Walton, K., Kleinman, K. P., Rifas-Shiman, S. L., Horton, N. J., Gillman, M. W., Field, A. E., . . . Haines, J. (2016). Secular trends in family dinner frequency among adolescents. *BMC Research Notes, 9*(1), 35.

4. Carroll, A. (2013, September 24). The decline of the family dinner (new book). *Huffington Post*. Retrieved from http://www.huffingtonpost.com/abigail-carroll/family-dinner_b_3977169.html.

5. Wolfson, J. A., & Bleich, S. N. (2015). Is cooking at home associated with better diet quality or weight-loss intention? *Public Health Nutrition, 18*(8), 1397–1406.

6. Center for Science in the Public Interest. (2013, March 28). *Kids' meals II: Obesity and poor nutrition on the menu.*

7. Reicks, M., Trofholz, A. C., Stang, J. S., & Laska, M. N. (2014). Impact of cooking and home food preparation interventions among adults: Outcomes and implications for future programs. *Journal of Nutrition Education and Behavior, 46*(4), 259–276. http://doi.org/10.1016/j.jneb.2014.02.001.

8. Condrasky, M., Graham, K., & Kamp, J. (2006). Cooking with a chef: An innovative program to improve mealtime practices and eating behaviors of caregivers of preschool children. *Journal of Nutrition Education and Behavior, 38*(5), 324–325.

9. Hersch, D., Perdue, L., Ambroz, T., & Boucher, J. L. (2014). The impact of cooking classes on food-related preferences, attitudes, and behaviors of school-aged children: A systematic review of the evidence, 2003–2014. *Preventing Chronic Disease, 11*, E193. http://doi.org/10.5888/pcd11.140267.

10. Ibid.

11. Musick, K., & Meier, A. (2012). Assessing causality and persistence in associations between family dinners and adolescent well-being. *Journal of Marriage and the Family, 74*(3), 476–493.

12. Meier, A., & Musick, K. (2014). Variation in associations between family dinners and adolescent well-being. *Journal of Marriage and the Family, 76*(1), 13–23. http://doi.org/10.1111/jomf.12079.

13. Harrison, M. E., Norris, M. L., Obeid, N., Fu, M., Weinstangel, H., & Sampson, M. (2015). Systematic review of the effects of family meal frequency on psychosocial outcomes in youth. *Canadian Family Physician, 61*(2), e96–e106.

14. Skeer, M. R., & Ballard, E. L. (2013). Are family meals as good for youth as we think they are? A review of the literature on family meals as they pertain to adolescent risk prevention. *Journal of Youth and Adolescence, 42*(7), 943–963.

Week 48: Have Strength in Yourself

1. Mann, M. M., Hosman, C. M., Schaalma, H. P., & De Vries, N. K. (2004). Self-esteem in a broad-spectrum approach for mental health promotion. *Health Education Research, 19*(4), 357–372.

2. Brummelman, E., Thomaes, S., Nelemans, S. A., De Castro, B. O., Overbeek, G., & Bushman, B. J. (2015). Origins of narcissism in children. *Proceedings of the National Academy of Sciences, 112*(12), 3659–3662.

3. van Scheppingen, M. A., Denissen, J., Chung, J., Tambs, K., & Bleidorn, W. (2017, August 10). Self-esteem and relationship satisfaction during the transition to motherhood. *Journal of Personality and Social Psychology.* doi: 10.1037/pspp0000156.

4. Allen, J. P., Chango, J., Szwedo, D., Schad, M., & Marston, E. (2012). Predictors of susceptibility to peer influence regarding substance use in adolescence. *Child Development, 83*(1), 337–350. http://doi.org/10.1111/j.1467-8624.2011.01682.x.

5. Briñol, P., Gascó, M., Petty, R. E., & Horcajo, J. (2013). Treating thoughts as material objects can increase or decrease their impact on evaluation. *Psychological Science, 24*(1), 41–47.

Week 49: Cultivate Emotional Intelligence

1. Salovey, P., & Mayer, J. D. (1990). Emotional intelligence. *Imagination, Cognition and Personality, 9*(3), 185–211.

2. Martins, A., Ramalho, N., & Morin, E. (2010). A comprehensive meta-analysis of the relationship between emotional intelligence and health. *Personality and Individual Differences, 49*(6), 554–564.

3. Chamorro-Premuzic, T., Bennett, E., & Furnham, A. (2007). The happy personality: Mediational role of trait emotional intelligence. *Personality and Individual Differences, 42*(8), 1633–1639.

4. Lopes, P. N., Grewal, D., Kadis, J., Gall, M., & Salovey, P. (2006). Evidence that emotional intelligence is related to job performance and affect and attitudes at work. *Psicothema, 18.*

5. Brackett, M. A., Rivers, S. E., & Salovey, P. (2011). Emotional intelligence: Implications for personal, social, academic, and workplace success. *Social and Personality Psychology Compass, 5*(1), 88–103.

6. See note 3 above.

7. Brackett, M. A., Palomera, R., Mojsa-Kaja, J., Reyes, M. R., & Salovey, P. (2010). Emotion regulation ability, burnout, and job satisfaction among British secondary-school teachers. *Psychology in the Schools, 47*(4), 406–417.

8. Graziano, P. A., Reavis, R. D., Keane, S. P., & Calkins, S. D. (2007). The role of emotion regulation in children's early academic success. *Journal of School Psychology, 45*(1), 3–19.

9. See note 2 above.

10. Eggum, N. D., Eisenberg, N., Kao, K., Spinrad, T. L., Bolnick, R., Hofer, C., . . . Fabricius, W. V. (2011). Emotion understanding, theory of mind, and prosocial orientation: Relations over time in early childhood. *The Journal of Positive Psychology, 6*(1), 4–16.

11. Brackett, M. A., Mayer, J. D., & Warner, R. M. (2004). Emotional intelligence and its relation to everyday behaviour. *Personality and Individual Differences, 36*(6), 1387–1402.

12. Chamorro-Premuzic, T. (2013, May 29). Can you really improve your emotional intelligence? *Harvard Business Review.*

13. Brackett, M. A., Warner, R. M., & Bosco, J. S. (2005). Emotional intelligence and relationship quality among couples. *Personal Relationships, 12*(2), 197–212.

14. Inside the teenage brain. (2002). *Frontline,* Public Broadcasting System.

15. Volling, B. L., McElwain, N. L., Notaro, P. C., & Herrera, C. (2002). Parents' emotional availability and infant emotional competence: Predictors of parent-infant attachment and emerging self-regulation. *Journal of Family Psychology, 16*(4), 447.

16. Ornaghi, V., Grazzani, I., Cherubin, E., Conte, E., & Piralli, F. (2015). "Let's talk about emotions!" The effect of conversational training on preschoolers' emotion comprehension and prosocial orientation. *Social Development, 24*(1), 166–183.

17. Tominey, S. L., O'Bryon, E. C., Rivers, S. E., & Shapses, S. (2017). Teaching emotional intelligence in early childhood. *Young Children, 72*(1).

18. Morris, A. S., Silk, J. S., Steinberg, L., Myers, S. S., & Robinson, L. R. (2007). The role of the family context in the development of emotion regulation. *Social Development, 16*(2), 361–388. http://doi.org/10.1111/j.1467-9507.2007.00389.x.

19. See note 12 above.

Week 50: Upgrade Your Medicine Cabinet

1. Fleming-Dutra, K. E., Hersh, A. L., Shapiro, D. J., Bartoces, M., Enns, E. A., File, T. M., . . . Lynfield, R. (2016). Prevalence of inappropriate antibiotic prescriptions among US ambulatory care visits, 2010–2011. *JAMA, 315*(17), 1864–1873.

2. Granado-Villar, D., Cunill-De Sautu, B., & Granados, A. (2012, November). Acute gastroenteritis. *Pediatrics in Review, 33*(11), 487–495.

3. Stanford Medicine News Center. (2009, November 17). *Common herbal medicine may prevent acetaminophen-related liver damage, says researcher.* Retrieved from https://med.stanford.edu/news/all-news/2009/11/common-herbal-medicine-may-prevent-acetaminophen-related-liver-damage-says-researcher.html.

4. Schillie, S. F., Shehab, N., Thomas, K. E., & Budnitz, D. S. (2009). Medication overdoses leading to emergency department visits among children. *American Journal of Preventive Medicine, 37*(3), 181–187.

5. Byington, C. L., Ampofo, K., Stockmann, C., Adler, F. R., Herbener, A., Miller, T., . . . Pavia, A. T. (2015). Community surveillance of respiratory viruses among families in the Utah Better Identification of Germs-Longitudinal Viral Epidemiology (BIG-LoVE) study. *Clinical Infectious Diseases, 61*(8), 1217–1224.

6. Davis, D. R., Epp, M. D., & Riordan, H. D. (2004). Changes in USDA food composition data for 43 garden crops, 1950 to 1999. *Journal of the American College of Nutrition, 23*(6), 669–682.

7. Walker, W. A. (2008). Mechanisms of action of probiotics. *Clinical Infectious Diseases, 46*(Supplement_2), S87–S91.

8. Weil, A. (n.d.). Homeopathic medicine. Retrieved from https://www.drweil.com/health-wellness/balanced-living/wellness-therapies/homeopathic-medicine/.

Week 51: Kick the Cow (not literally)

1. Bentley, J., & Kantor, L. (2016). Food availability (per capita) data system. Economic Research Service, United States Department of Agriculture. Retrieved from https://www.ers.usda.gov/data-products/food-availability-per-capita-data-system.

2. Welsh, J. A., Sharma, A., Cunningham, S. A., & Vos, M. B. (2011). Consumption of added sugars and indicators of cardiovascular disease risk among US adolescents. *Circulation, 123*(3), 249–257.

3. Yang, Q., Zhang, Z., Gregg, E. W., Flanders, W. D., Merritt, R., & Hu, F. B. (2014). Added sugar intake and cardiovascular diseases mortality among US adults. *JAMA Internal Medicine, 174*(4), 516–524.

4. Chen, M., Li, Y., Sun, Q., Pan, A., Manson, J. E., Rexrode, K. M., . . . Hu, F. B. (2016). Dairy fat and risk of cardiovascular disease in 3 cohorts of US adults. *American Journal of Clinical Nutrition, 104*(5), 1209–1217.

5. Feskanich, D., Willett, W. C., & Colditz, G. A. (2003). Calcium, vitamin D, milk consumption, and hip fractures: A prospective study among postmenopausal women. *American Journal of Clinical Nutrition, 77*(2), 504–511.

6. Fenton, T. R., & Hanley, D. A. (2006). Calcium, dairy products, and bone health in children and young adults: An inaccurate conclusion. *Pediatrics, 117*(1), 259–260.

7. Lanou, A. J., & Barnard, N. D. (2006). Calcium, dairy products, and bone health in children and young adults: An inaccurate conclusion: In reply. *Pediatrics, 117*(1), 260–261.

8. Sonneville, K. R., Gordon, C. M., Kocher, M. S., Pierce, L. M., Ramappa, A., & Field, A. E. (2012). Vitamin D, calcium, and dairy intakes and stress fractures among female adolescents. *Archives of Pediatrics & Adolescent Medicine, 166*(7), 595–600.

9. Berkey, C. S., Rockett, H. R., Willett, W. C., & Colditz, G. A. (2005). Milk, dairy fat, dietary calcium, and weight gain: A longitudinal study of adolescents. *Archives of Pediatrics & Adolescent Medicine, 159*(6), 543–550.

Week 52: Go Global

1. Marian, V., & Shook, A. (2012, September). The cognitive benefits of being bilingual. In W. Donway (Ed.), *Cerebrum: The Dana forum on brain science* (Vol. 2012). Collingdale, PA: Diane Publishing.

2. Tadmor, C. T., Galinsky, A. D., & Maddux, W. W. (2012, September). Getting the most out of living abroad: Biculturalism and integrative complexity as key drivers of creative and professional success. *Journal of Personality and Social Psychology, 103*(3), 520–42. doi: 10.1037/a0029360.

3. American Council on the Teaching of Foreign Languages (ACTFL). (n.d.). References for cognitive question: There is evidence that early language learning improves cognitive abilities. Retrieved from https://www.actfl.org/advocacy/what-the -research-shows/references-cognitive.

4. See note 2 above.

5. See note 1 above.

6. See note 2 above.

7. Leung, A. K. Y., Maddux, W. W., Galinsky, A. D., & Chiu, C. Y. (2008). Multicultural experience enhances creativity: The when and how. *American Psychologist, 63*(3), 169.

8. Cheng, E. (2017, April 30). *Here's why earnings are so outstanding even though the US economy is barely growing.* Market Insider, CNBC. Retrieved from https://www.cnbc .com/2017/04/30/heres-why-earnings-are-so-outstanding-even-while-the-us -economy-is-barely-growing.html.

9. U.S. Department of State. (2016). J-1 Visa Exchange Visitor Program, Participant and Sponsor Totals, Secondary School 2016. Retrieved from https://j1visa.state.gov/basics /facts-and-figures/.

Tools and Resources

1. Campbell, E. (2016, November 8). Three activities to help students deepen their gratitude. *Greater Good.* Retrieved from http://greatergood.berkeley.edu/article/item /three_activities_to_help_students_deepen_their_gratitude.

ACKNOWLEDGMENTS

Thank you to Meg Thompson and Sandy Hodgman for being in our corner. Thank you to everyone at Chronicle who dedicated hours to making this book a reality.

To the sisterhood of mothers that surrounds each of us with love, light, a listening ear, and judgement-free support every day, especially when we need it most. We would not be here without you. You have lifted us up and inspired us to share the collective knowledge of our parenting journeys in this book. We hope the research and tips provided do for you what they have done for us—ignite your passion and commitment to raising a happy, healthy family.

To the fathers who envelop us with love, compassion, and strength—your steadfast commitment to raising happy, healthy children (no matter how unconventional the approach may be) is truly amazing.

— Danielle and Brett

To my dear co-author, Brett, I am forever grateful for the chance you took on me in writing this book with you. Your patience, eloquence, and unrivalled time management skills made this book what it is today. I look forward to our next adventure together!

— Danielle

To my sweet friend and co-author, Danielle, you are amazing. I always stand in awe of all that you are and do. I'm so very proud of you for all that you have accomplished with this book. Your dedication, patience (with me especially), and your commitment have been beyond what I ever imagined. I can't wait to see what else the future holds for you!

— Brett

INDEX

associated with lower risk of breast cancer and heart disease. Other oils to consider include avocado oil, hemp seed oil, macadamia nut oil, sesame oil, walnut oil, and, of course, extra-virgin olive oil.

LOAD UP ON SEEDS   Many types of seeds are rich in healthy fats, protein, vitamins, and minerals. Plus, with the recent growth in nut allergies, seeds are a safe and healthy alternative for all children.

TYPE OF SEED	NUTRITIONAL BENEFITS	HOW TO EAT THEM
Chia	High in omega-3 fats and fiber; packed with calcium, magnesium, and phosphorus, all good for bone health	Atop salads and oatmeal; make a pudding or thicken soup
Pumpkin (with or without shells)	High in polyunsaturated fat and iron (23 percent of daily recommended value for adults), magnesium, copper, and zinc	Alone, in trail mix, atop salads or veggies
Sesame	Highly nutritious source of calcium, magnesium, iron, zinc, and manganese	Atop salads, stir-fry dishes, and cooked veggies; grind 5 parts sesame seeds with 1 part Celtic sea salt to create "gomashio," a salt alternative
Sunflower	Excellent source of monounsaturated fat, vitamin E, copper, selenium, and vitamin B1 (thiamine)	In trail mix or atop salads, or pureed to create sunbutter, a nut butter alternative

GO NUTS   Like seeds, nuts are also loaded with high-quality fats, protein, vitamins, and minerals. You can eat them alone or as part of trail mix. Other options include pureed into nut butter, atop salads and vegetable dishes, baked in desserts and muffins, soaked and strained into milk, or ground up and used as flour. Here are a few highly nutritious favorites:

Expeller-pressing is a chemical-free process that extracts oil from nuts or seeds by crushing them with extreme pressure at various temperatures. Although the expeller-pressed oils are not treated with hexane during the expeller pressing process, note that they may be treated with hexane afterward to extract more of the remaining oil.

When you shop for oils, look for those that are unrefined, cold-pressed, or expeller-pressed.

Sautéing/pan frying Contrary to popular practice, not all oil is appropriate for high-heat cooking. For example, because of its prevalence in our culture, extra-virgin olive oil is commonly used with heat that is too high for safe consumption. If you overheat oil, you will see it smoking in the pan and notice a change in smell. When this happens, dump the oil, wipe the pan, and start with fresh oil on a lower heat setting.

Baking Any oil that can be heated on the stovetop can also be used in baking. Coconut oil has gained much popularity recently and for good reason. Though it is a saturated fat, coconut oil is high in lauric acid, an anti-inflammatory compound, and is used by the body as energy more quickly than other fats. Avocado oil has minimal flavor and can easily be used in baking, though it is more expensive than other baking oils. Extra-virgin olive oil has a stronger flavor and usually works best in more savory baked goods. Finally, unrefined red palm oil has a slightly sweet buttery flavor and is loaded with many antioxidants and vitamins. That said, not all palm oil is created equal. Be sure to choose unrefined, sustainably cultivated red palm oil that maintains its red color—otherwise the oil has been highly processed and is missing most health benefits.

Dressings Store-bought salad dressings are often loaded with additives and unhealthy ingredients, especially poor-quality oils. Upgrade dressings for salads and vegetable dipping by adding in nutrient-dense oils. Flaxseed oil, one of the richest sources of plant-based omega-3 fat, has a nutty flavor and is also full of lignans, a polyphenol, or plant compound,